DYNAMIC HEALTH RESTORATION

A Guide for Modern Times

Dr. Brooke Heather

AuthorHouse™
1663 Liberty Drive
Bloomington, IN 47403
www.authorhouse.com
Phone: 833-262-8899

Because of the dynamic nature of the Internet, any web addresses or links contained in this book may have changed since publication and may no longer be valid. The views expressed in this work are solely those of the author and do not necessarily reflect the views of the publisher, and the publisher hereby disclaims any responsibility for them.

Any people depicted in stock imagery provided by Getty Images are models, and such images are being used for illustrative purposes only.
Certain stock imagery © Getty Images.

This book is printed on acid-free paper.

ISBN: 978-1-6655-0659-5 (sc)
ISBN: 978-1-6655-0660-1 (e)

Print information available on the last page.

Published by AuthorHouse 02/23/2022

authorHOUSE®

Contents

Acknowledgements

There is simply nothing better to me in my life at this time than the loving support as well as significant assistance in the production of this book than that of which my amazingly supportive husband Aryan Riener has provided me. Words cannot do justice to the immense gratitude I have for you, your family and our awesome combined family. How blessed I feel to have true unconditional love and companionship in my life.

Thanks to all the people who took a look at this project in its many forms as it evolved, even before the vision of it becoming a book, and helped with editing: Heidi Christy, Pricilla Boward, Akasha Reiner and Jonnie Bradley with special thanks to your contributions to the amazing summary of the book. Additionally, the marvelous and kind review by Professor DA Cole.

Illustration design of the diagrams and book cover was a breeze working with Jenavieve Hawks, many thanks!

I make a special dedication of this book to my two beautiful daughters that are brave souls to have chosen to incarnate during these times. May their lives be blessed, protected and used for good; I pray. My soul acknowledges you both as precious souls, serving a higher purpose. May strength and remembrance of who you are and what this important purpose you serve be known to you and culminate soon.

Introduction

Do you get confused and overwhelmed sometimes, by how much information is out there on health and wellness? There is no doubt, conflicting information is everywhere. Now is the time to take control of your health. It is my aspiration to empower you with a reliable guide based on original tried and true traditional methods of self-healing. Old wisdom ways are rediscovered and simplified into manageable steps. The personalized methods, you can start implementing to turn your health around and maintain wellness. The goal is to avoid unwanted healthcare expenses.

You may have been in a place of discouragement following healthcare appointments and leave more confused than before. This guide includes a wide variety of valuable information to address acute illness and how to rule out dangerous gastrointestinal conditions. Specializing in digestive health, I have found this to be an important area to dial in. You will discover information for your family with a helpful rule-out method of how to know when to seek more professional expertise.

I will first demystify nutritional supplementation before taking you through the most needed nutrients for your body to regenerate. Through clinical practice, there are distinct deficiencies in the masses that I will outline. I will clarify food groups then we will voyage through how to personalize your diet to best fit your individual needs. I provide ideas of how to practically organize your meals in order to get all those nutrients from foods and whole food supplementation (very different from chemical isolates, synthetically made). Most importantly, I detail digestion-promoting practices and correct food combining awareness, critical in gaining and maintaining health. Learn about "anti-nutrients," which may surprise you. See samples of properly combined meals and drive home the principles throughout the diagrams with the Vital Food Plan guidelines. Learn about emotional eating and do the corresponding inner work to resolve the cause. Everything from ridding yourself of parasites to weight loss and keys to self-assessment, both psycho-spiritually and physically, are all provided in this one-of-a-kind book.

Healing doesn't begin with the physical acts we do, such as a change in diet. The beginning of a regenerative process begins in the energy body and is supported greatly through wholesome foods. Wholesome foods cleanse and nourish the body. Once we take the steps to balance the energy that sustains life in our bodies, we have the potential to achieve robust health. A large portion of this book is dedicated to psycho-spiritual-socio-emotional wellbeing.

The origin of this book began as a short guide for my clients, which I used to instruct them about how to properly combine foods for ideal digestion and modify their lifestyle to eliminate toxins. It has now morphed into a comprehensive manual with assessment keys used clinically. I want you to have this knowledge and access it for yourself and family. This work is what makes the world a better, purer and a healthier place with every reader that implements the content.

My passion for this work began with the conception of my first child, now over sixteen years ago. I had strong intuition and belonged to a family that fostered that in me. I remember the strong feelings intuitively guiding me away from the use of any product with harmful chemicals. There were not health food stores or "organic" produce back then, at least not for this Wyoming girl. I knew I had to clean up my diet and up my nutrition. Some short time after I did, I noticed my once awful nails with deep ridges that would also peel off in layers turned beautiful, smooth and strong. My frizzy straight hair I once hated became so much healthier looking. Prior to this, it was suggested to me that I go to a salon for weekly conditioner treatments because my hair was so unhealthy. My skin cleared up and I felt more energetic than ever. I had always been a low energy person. I had skin rashes on and off all my life. In just the short time of my pregnancy, all this was 100% better. A large portion of this major transition from obviously being nutritionally depleted to vibrant and clear of physical manifestations of deficiencies had to have been the fact that I was given purpose for the first time in my life with the coming of my son. Not that I was depressed by any means but something about conceiving him brought a spark to life I'll never forget and forever hold dear. After his birth I began my education as I raised him. I purchased a Biofeedback medical device. I did studies from home, earning the title of Certified Holistic Health Practitioner while I practiced as a Biofeedback technician and later Specialist. I became intrigued with Neuroscience and what promise the testing of neurotransmitters and hormones could provide as a window into my clients' health. I graduated with a double Masters in Traditional Naturopathy and Integrative Medicine in 2008, thus allowing me to enroll in post grad trainings such as Functional Diagnostic Medicine and my many other certifications and trainings in various areas. I have learned that the testing of all the chemicals we can test for in the body is only one portion of a large puzzle. Ancient medical systems, through their very different forms of evaluations, show us what the body needs in a completely holistic manner. This doesn't negate modern testing, as information is always helpful, but information itself does not cure illnesses. Sadly, our modern allopathic medical model fails to direct patients to the methods which would restore health. It is my hope to bridge that gap of individuals who fit the above demographic by providing preventative as well as curative methods of restoring wellbeing as much as possible. I hope you take the time to immerse yourself in the following pages and do the inner work as well. As with any program, it is best to team up with other like-minded individuals. This is especially important as your live-in family is typically not as supportive as much as you need. With this I must give thanks to my tribe and all those that have participated in the study I conducted in completion of my Doctorate in Alternative Medicine.

Epigenetics vs. Genetics

I often hear "Oh, it's genetic," when it comes to reproductive issues involving the glands (which are responsible for producing hormones) or heart disease, anemias, and other chronic conditions. This term or the way it is often spoken implies a sense of complacency. But your genes are not your fate! Genetic flaws or mutations can occur from genetically modified organisms (GMOs) and not having the building blocks—that is, proteins. You do not need to consume more meat to acquire these building blocks. Proteins are in all foods. You do, however, need to find out what you are deficient in and to be sure you are fully digesting your food. First, find the cause. *Genetic inheritance* is rarely an excuse for the acceptance of a condition. If you feel you need more guidance than this book can provide, arrange to assess causes during an office visit or phone consultation. Second, identify the materials you should provide the body so it can do the work of repair. The body is designed for repair, so believe that it can—but not with drugs, as they do not heal, and not with synthetic vitamins. I will be very specific about distinguishing between healing substances to use as supplements and chemicals that mimic the purpose of a drug merely to change symptoms, but not to heal.

Avoiding genetically modified foods will greatly increase the integrity of your cells, therefore the tissues that make up organs and every system of your body. A condition involving a system that is seen throughout a lineage, as with *genetic* disorders, is a nutritional deficiency that must be addressed with the supplementation of whole food concentrates; with a specialized therapeutic substance called PMG therapy (discussed later) for the duration of one's lifespan in this case.

Skepticism causes us to question how we could be "vitamin C" deficient, for example. Vitamin C, commonly known as ascorbic acid, is not the true full-spectrum nutrient in its complexity intended for our bodies as nutrition. Our system is not designed to take in chemical isolates and turn them into a usable form. Consumption of over the counter (OTC) supplements and at times supplements given or recommended by healthcare professionals (unknowingly sourced from GMO corn, or petroleum byproducts), causes further imbalance and deficiency. **Taking supplements that are isolated chemicals is only creating a deficiency in the other parts of the dynamic nutrient you are intending to provide your body with**.

Many of you reading this are anti Big Pharma, or want to get off the band wagon because you are wise enough to know that pharmaceuticals are not healing you and have negative effects. Stay with me through this concept of comparison to the nutritional supplement industry below. I hope to make a lasting impression with this information. The whole idea of a medication is to address the symptoms of a person. Essentially, the use of pharmaceuticals is to change the way the person's experience or what I call "symptom picture." This is a dangerous game, as the root issues are not being supported in a way that induce healing, rather the disease process continues. The body merely finds a different channel of manifesting the disorder. Now here is the "Wow!"— Similarly, we seek supplementation of so-called nutrition to improve health. You purchase a supplement with an impressive list in the nutritional facts and trust that it is good. This is the hopeful side of you looking through rose-colored glasses. You really want it to be good for you, so you perceive that it is. You might hear good things about the brand, about it being "pure' or "quality" sourced. The truth is, these are copies of vitamins, that Dr. Ulan states as "built wrong from cancerous substance." What he is saying here is that the pharmaceutical companies own the rights to the majority of the synthetically made vitamins. Furthermore, many of the supplement companies themselves are owned by pharmaceutical companies. Because of marketing, you may believe you are replacing missing nutrients with certain products when in reality only whole foods can provide complete nutrition.

Practitioners practicing nutrition may not even know that they are in fact practicing orthomolecular medicine – mega dosing. It is bypassing the nervous system and correct pathways of regenerative healing, unlike the body so wisely does with the raw materials (if supplied), and simply changes the physiology in order to change the symptoms. Changing symptoms does not equate to healing or truly getting better.

I will continue the point I am making about supplementation using the example of vitamin C because it remains one of the most over-dosed, misunderstood substances the general public is misinformed about. Real vitamin C, as nature intended for our consumption, has many counter parts, some likely unknown. You can't simply take vitamin C for vascular wall integrity along with the ever-so-common prescribed baby aspirin per day and expect anything *other than further deterioration of the lumen, or lining of the vascular walls*. Non-steroidal anti-inflammatories such as aspirin destroy the over 60,000 miles of vessels, veins, arteries and capillaries, compromising our cardiovascular system. What is really needed is what I refer to as the anti-stroke factor, called vitamin P, also referred to as bioflavonoids. These are constituents you may have heard of in the last few years. They are added to many vitamin C products to increase effectiveness.

This is just one example of other known counterparts that should comprise vitamin C as a complex. I use this misunderstood quasi-vitamin as an example both to distinguish the difference between a true nutrient found in nature verses a chemical isolate. As "pure" as they may be with their expensive price tag, pure in this sense is used merely to denote the absence of any other constituent. Many chemical isolates are derived from GMO sources, such as ascorbic acid is made from corn syrup and vitamin Bs from coal, tar and petroleum. Alternately, the collagen producing vitamin C complex, such as in the product Cyruta, made from the leaves of the buckwheat plant, is natures best anti-stroke and tissue repair "Vitamin C" product. **As you will come to see, isolation of constituents is not what heals the body. Nor does it imbue healing qualities like nature-made complex foods and herbs do**.

I do not recommend anything other than whole food sources of supplementation. Humans cannot replicate the intricate work of nature and I highly advise NOT to mega-dose! This concept applies to all nutrients/vitamins. If you are taking supplements that have a list with measured out amounts in "mg" (milligrams) or otherwise, you are inoculating your system with chemical isolates that are likely contributing to a variety of other deficiencies and imbalances in the cofactors (explained more in-depth later) of the very nutrient you had intended to increase with supplementation. This is a system of robbing Peter to pay Paul. How do you suppose you can correct the deficiency you created with your supplementation of isolated chemicals that drained your body of the cofactors when those cofactors have not been synthesized yet? You can't simply go out and buy what you are lacking. Additionally, these cofactors to the vitamins in supplements are often depleted in foods. Are you depressed yet? Speaking of which, take your vitamin D! Or wait, does this above concept apply to chemicals (referred to as nutrients) across the board? The ever so popular vitamin D many people are mega dosing with, and medical doctors are now also recommending, is a hormone-like chemical. Not realizing that it creates calcium starvation in the tissues when taken out of proportion with its counterparts. If muscle cramps occur, it is seen as a separate issue. You might pop some magnesium for the leg cramps when in fact the cramping of muscles in this case is caused by the calcium starvation. Vitamin D prevents calcium from being utilized within the tissues of the body, so it remains in the blood. Calcium sustained in the blood causes a whole host of problems. In contrast, vitamin D naturally in foods causes uptake of calcium by the tissues because the fatty acids remain in proportion to the vitamin D. Tissues can become calcium deprived resulting in leg cramps or charley horses and may result in excessive bleeding and hemorrhaging. You see, everything in nature maintains ideal ratios of nutrients. The imbalance in foods occurs with depleted soils and toxicity in the environment. Regardless, sourcing your food from the highest possible growing conditions is the aim. Additionally, whole food supplements, professionally recommended, is the only way to do it if you are going to do so with the intent to come into balance.

Most people are using what they would call vitamins, minerals or nutrients with the mindset that mimics the pharmaceutical mythology: take x for condition A, take y for condition B and so on. How many different symptoms do you have? Find out how your symptoms correlate with body systems with a quick survey (see resources in the back of book).

Affordable healthcare, to me, means efficient, yet thorough assessment of the areas that need strengthened or repaired and providing the tools to restore the body's wholeness. Nothing can do this but the innate intelligence of the body having the raw materials to do so.

Herbs are an important addition to any healing endeavor and especially helpful to assist in the mental/emotional harmony, brought on with the herb best suitable for your constitution. Furthermore, herbs that are wild crafted provide the most natural environment possible for the health of the plant. It is important to work with a health professional (HP) well trained in herbology and not to self-administer herbs beyond the use of mild herbal teas. Herbs have properties such as "warming" or "cooling," for example, that can push someone constitutionally "too warm" or "too cold" further into their condition, undermining the intent. It is simply not wise to use herbs without knowing a great deal about your constitution and the herb considered before use. Furthermore, as much as there are wonderful books out there on the benefit herbs provide, I have not come across one that can direct you adequately on personalized methodology and proper administration of an herb. It's wonderful to educate yourself on the wondrous benefits herbs provide us and maybe in a future book I will make a list of safe-for-most herbs for home use. For example, this would include most herbs we use as spices along with aloe, dandelion and Gotu Kola. In the selection of herbs, a truly holistic approach in making a recommendation, not only considers underlying root causes of the presenting condition, but also what the physical body type of the person is that the herbs are being recommended for. Additionally, the person's personality/temperament can play a role in the selection of specific herbs. There are not many herbs that I can speak freely of without feeling like I would want to assess a person before recommending the herb. However, in this case, speaking on the topic of genetics, I will introduce burdock as it is said to correct damage done by the ingestion of genetically modified organisms or GMO's. With this you will see the power that herbs contain, yet one must remember they are all different and possess more than seventy different therapeutic properties, each with their own set of combinations.

Burdock is safe for pregnancy and most everyone. However, there have been cases of allergic reactions. As with any use of herbs for the first time, start out slow and with a low dose. Reactions can happen with anything new. The physical restorative aspect of burdock involves its fantastic blood cleansing quality. I think of it as going around gathering the old and unwanted to make way for the new. In the sense of blood, burdock is a vulnerary herb, meaning it promotes healing. It is also antineoplastic which destroys cancer cells and inhibits the growth of tumors. Now that is an effective blood cleanser; more like a cellular revitalizer (we just don't have a term for that yet in herbology). Many Native American tribes used this root for a variety of diseases and skin conditions. The Chinese use it to balance blood sugar and hormones. As you can imagine, it must curb inflammation having these above listed qualities. Any time we can put out the fire of inflammation within our system our body can begin the healing work. A professional line I recommend due to potency and guaranteed quality is from MediHerb and only distributed through professionals (please do not purchase off Amazon, it is illegal for it to be sold through that avenue and has potential to be a scam). It is a combination product. It is especially good for healing of the gut, having slippery elm in the formula. Slippery elm is one of the best nutritive herbs and as a first baby food. It is soothing and protective to the lining of the intestines. Being a nutritive and mucilant it helps heal any gastrointestinal conditions. Burdock Complex is used in my cancer care protocol to modulate the immune system, clear toxins, support healthy elimination and mucosal membranes and healthy blood. I also like to use this formula during annual cleanses and is recommended as maintenance for certain genetic or hereditary tendencies.

Epigenetics is taking control over gene expression by controlling the environment. Each gene has the potential to create up to 2000 varieties of protein. This regenerative process depends upon multiple factors. The variables that influence genetic expression are environmental as well as mental/emotional.

25,000 genes generate 100,000 proteins

Energy is not defined *simply* as a level of feeling or an expression of life but rather a vital life force; a vibrational state. The below suggestions can become rituals used to increase the quality of your life, thus resulting in healthier gene expression.

TIPS FOR INCREASING VITALITY:

- Massage with essential oil blend (diluted in a carrier oil of course).
- Foot bath with sea salts and essential oils— an energizing, grounding, and regenerative therapy (see recipe in Chapter "Laws of Nature").
- Brush teeth with essential oils (Oral Oil). The teeth are connected to the organs and meridians. The use of essential oil orally increases stimulation of the entire body and promotes healthy digestion and immunity. Consult with us about a customized blend. You want to base your essential oil choice on your Ayurvedic Dosha which will be discussed later.
- Wear all-natural clothing, like organic cotton or wool next to the skin.

Decline of Health

1. Cellular insufficiency (inadequate conversion of food into energy)
2. Organ insufficiency (poor digestion and malabsorption)
3. Insufficient detoxification/elimination (toxic buildup in tissues and cells)
4. Further impaired cellular function
5. Inability to repair and rebuild body tissue
6. Organ, gland, and systemic dysfunction
7. Sub clinical symptoms
8. Clinical symptoms and disease

For more information, see *The Causes of Disorder* below.

The Organic Investment

Economics 101 says it's better to spend a lot for something than a little for nothing! If you keep the honest farmer in business while investing more in your family's health and the future generation, only then will a society be sustainable!

What is the difference in produce? Is it worth the extra cost? At times organic can be double or three times the amount of conventionally grown produce! I don't even look at the empty harvest. In all reality, is it truly **empty**, and not only void of nutritional content but also containing harmful hormone disrupting chemicals? Metabolic mayhem is a direct result of the glyphosate (RoundUp™) exposure. RoundUp™ ready crops (mainly corn, canola, oats, wheat, soy and sugar beets) are sprayed to ripen the crop right before harvest. Additionally, we have exposure to this carcinogenic toxin through our cotton clothing and in the air we breathe via the ethanol fuel. My point is that glyphosate exposure is unavoidable so limiting consumption of it can be prioritized.

Reasons to shop organic, local and/or grow your own produce:

- To avoid the estrogenic (mimics estrogen; too much causes cancer, obesity, etc.) effects of pesticides and other toxins.
- More nutritional value equating to longevity in the integrity of our cells (health).
- To keep local/small businesses practicing sustainable farming in business! The cost of organic food may come down as support increases.
- The more demand there is for healthier options, the more we preserve Mother Earth and the integrity of all living beings supported on our planet.
- When you consume healthy animal products, you receive information not only about the health of that animal, but the status of the foods from which it ate and the soil it grew in! Your dietary choices change the way your genes function!

Pointers:

- Stay abreast the Environmental Working Group (EWG) "Dirty Dozen" list. It includes the top twelve fruits and vegetables found to have the highest amount of pesticide residue.
- Within the *Metabolic Regulatory Food Chart*, produce highlighted in green, should be prioritized as foods to purchase organically according to the EWG research. This chart is handy to use as a shopping list.

Doctors of the Past

"Not a single incidence of cancer among the natives subsiding on their traditional foods," one American medical doctor reported. He lived among the Eskimos and northern Indians for thirty-five years and observed that when illness began it was only with the introduction of "white man's" food. When tuberculosis and other disorders prevailed, the doctor would send them back to their native villages and they would recover! Dr. Westin discovered the "sacred foods" of primitive cultures by living with them and observing how the food was grown and prepared. He reports case after case of his findings in his book <u>Nutritional and Physical Degeneration.</u>

Traditional diets across the world contained animal organs as well as meat, substantial fat, and various forms of fermented foods and beverages. These foods provided abundant nutrients that are greatly lacking in the Standard American Diet (SAD).

Vegetarianism

While I can understand and do agree with many of the reasons why one would choose to be a vegetarian, I feel there are hurdles to overcome. Although it can be done, to be a vegetarian, one must be diligent and almost perfect with their diet in order to be well nourished. It is especially difficult to get enough fat-soluble vitamins. I also have observed that vegetarians don't avoid the yummy, addicting, convenient comfort foodstuff of breads, baked goods and pastas. Often, when your body is starved for nutrition these are the very cravings one has and are most difficult to not indulged upon.

Taken for face value, every sign of health found through a look at the tongue, nails, skin and hair of vegetarians is telling of depletion. This is a finding more so in vegetarians than in those who are not. The problem of over-consumption of the above listed foodstuff is common among all economically developed demographics. The difference is in the deficiency of fat-soluble vitamins, particularly A, critical for what some would call anti-aging. In effect, "anti-aging" is accurate in that it denotes the regenerative, life-sustaining capacity of our cells. Zinc and vitamin A work hand in hand. Zinc deficiency can be due to the over-consumption of sugar and carbs. Most Americans and industrialized nations are inflicted with this poor dietary custom. Furthermore, think about the foods that provide the best sources of zinc... organ meats, eggs, dark green leafy greens (which, dependent on source may or may not contain adequate amounts of nutrients) and then come nuts, seeds and grains, all which if not taken from their raw source and soaked or sprouted, are doing the body virtually no good nutritionally only providing the fat and fiber. So, as you can imagine the general population of meat-consuming individuals being zinc deficient due to the above outlined scenario, how much more-so would the vegetarian be, being that they avoid the top three sources for zinc? The average adult would have to consume about five eggs per day to obtain the *minimum* amount of recommended daily value in much needed zinc. As you may be aware, children may require even more nutrients than an adult while they are developing. As with any injury or need for healing, known or unknown, additional zinc along with other nutrients and proteins are required for the body to heal adequately.

The more legumes, nuts, seeds and grains you consume (that are not soaked or sprouted) the more *micronutrients you will need to supplement with. The lectins in these foods bind to the trace minerals making them unavailable for nutrient absorption.

*Organically Bound Minerals is a good whole food supplement for vegetarians although I would highly recommend supplementing with Trace Minerals B12 and the other non-vegetarian supplements to get raw high-quality protein with all the amino acids.

A great supplement regimen for someone that prefers to eat vegetarian would consist of Collagen C, Cataplex A, Zinc Liver Chelate, Trace Minerals B12 and Symplex M or F (male or female) for starters.

The endocrine system is the first to be depleted with inadequate protein (amino acids). The endocrine system comprises the glands (thyroid, adrenal, pituitary, hypothalamus, gonads, etc.) that synthesize hormones. With the breakdown of this system, or any organ or muscle for that matter begins to deteriorate. The body needs all twenty-two amino acids available so that it is not having to rob the muscles and other storehouses of amino acids. This deterioration, or breakdown, of the body's tissue can be avoided if not malnourished.

I will give just one example of an amino acid that is a prevalent deficiency that is very hard to get through the diet, and especially for vegetarians due to the fact the only significant sources are from meat and eggs but only in their raw form. This amino acid is called glutamine. It is called a conditionally essential amino acid. This means the body cannot make as much as it requires under states of stress and/or injury. Who doesn't have injuries or an increased state of stress from time to time? It is then easy to reason that this amino acid, glutamine, can become depleted quite readily. It is the most abundant amino acid contained in the blood and brain with high concentrations found in the liver, stomach. About 60% of the total glutamine stores are concentrated in the skeletal muscles and when the body requires the amino acid, it is released into the bloodstream where it is transported to the tissue in need (Birkner). The immune cells require the most demand for glutamine. It is said that glutamine is the most important nutrient for the intestinal tract (Birkner).

Personally, I enjoy eating vegetarian ninety percent of the time. However, I supplement with glandulars (animal glands/tissue for therapeutic purposes). I like the Eastern philosophy or Vedic principle of non-violence and taking only what you need, and I also know that my body needs the support and quality proteins along with mega nutrient content that animal glands provide because of the amount of stress I undergo. Due to this stress beyond my control, I see the supplementation of glandulars in the form of PMG's as a preventative measure against auto-immune conditions that could otherwise be festering. I trust in the sourcing/quality of Standard Process' glandular products from animals that otherwise would have been wasted. I consider it part of the cycle of life and aim to have a balanced approach. I must point out that animals die, their glands are wasted in the typical muscle meats sold. I find this disturbing un-natural as all primitive diets utilized the whole animal. The cycle of life applied here lends credence to the idea of both plant and animal kingdoms being available medicinally to utilize with gratitude and great regard. We humans have the means to manage our environment. We don't simple live in it like animals, rather we tend to it (or have the ability to). I intend, when I pass, to have my ashes spread in our garden compost; "back to dust." "Made from salt and dust," I return to Mother Earth.

Processed at low temperatures, considered "raw" in the processing, glandulars provide the peptides, RNA and quality proteins needed to feed the glands of my body adequately. I believe it is a smart and quite convenient way to supplement with the glandulars to be sure I am getting quality protein (raw, undenatured). Glandulars, are instrumental in the regulation of our glands. Protomorphogins or PMG's translates into "change over time" meaning taking the substance builds up the gland of the Protomorphogin/PMG ingested i.e., the PMG supplementation of the thyroid rebuilds the thyroid, the PMG for the heart builds and regulates the heart, the spleen, liver and so on. There is a PMG for virtually every organ and gland also the bone PMG for the balancing of minerals in the body, for the immune system and healing of bones themselves and cavities of the teeth. PMG's are the best form of glandulars and safe to take long-term. PMG's differ from whole desiccated glands that are not intended for use over three months' time. Because glands manufacture compounds called hormones which set off a whole cascade of chemical reactions within our body, it is called PMG Therapy to supplement with this portion of the gland, protomorphogin (PMG) is supplemented over a long-term.

PMG Therapy is a form of medicine and very effective when needed. Furthermore, I believe PMG Therapy shouldn't be disregarded for ethical reasons which is a good reason to be vegetarian on the topic of the treatment of the animals. Because there are good quality sources of the animals to which the glands are used, this should be the focal point. Due to our depleted soils producing nutritionally out-of-proportion crops, I find it even more important to supplement with glanulars as a body (human or animal) strives to maintain the vital organs and glands of proper compositions so that they continue to function optimally. My point being, even though an animal's food source is depleted, the body does what it can to maintain the integrity of its vital systems, even at the cost of robbing the bones. This is why we are at an ever-increasing rate of osteoporosis in the U.S.

Some individuals believe there are moral and spiritual reasons for being a vegetarian. I would have to agree that there is a higher vibration in solely consuming a plant-based diet and therefore, I regard PMG Therapy as medicine from finite animals. So, unless you have zero stress depleting your reserves of minerals and an excellent diet with absolutely no symptoms, I see supplementation necessary. Organ meats pack a punch when it comes to nutritional content *with* the added benefit of PMG Therapy (only through a healthcare provider that can recommend you Standard Process supplements. They are the only glandular that does not heat the material).

As stated in *Heal with Amino Acids and Nutrients:* If you remove the water and fat from the body, amino acids comprise the remaining 75%. Amino acids are referred to as the building blocks of life because all protein is made up of amino acids that are responsible for all the functions we think of our nervous system governing. This includes emotional responses and muscle movement. The brain's billions of neurons conduct communications via neurotransmitters (neuro-hormones) carrying signals of sensation.

The Cholesterol Riddle

What is something many people call "bad," that is produced by the body, and is essential for digestion? A lipid molecule called *cholesterol*. Any need in the body for healing places a demand on the body that increases endogenous levels of cholesterol because it is a "healing molecule." It comes to the rescue, repairing tissues in need of healing. This means if you're recovering from something and your body is in "heal mode," you may test higher than normal for cholesterol. As with everything else, it's the balance between the two primary lipoproteins that matter; not the value of total cholesterol. This is detailed below, and I recommend being informed of the ratio and doing the calculation rather than relying of your physician. You must remember, they are trained to sell pharmaceuticals. Your physician is also educated about the "ideal levels" by the pharmaceutical company's representatives (sales reps) and their agenda.

As with all other nutrients, the blood carries cholesterol throughout the body to nourish the tissues. Bound with a protein and in this form traveling in the blood, the compound is called a lipoprotein. The two lipoproteins of focus are high-density lipoproteins (HDL) and low-density lipoproteins (LDL). You've heard of LDL referred to as "the bad type of cholesterol." Low-density lipoprotein (LDL) binds most of the protein in the body and carries cholesterol from the liver to the cells throughout the body. High-density lipoprotein (HDL) gathers cholesterol from the blood vessels and tissues and carries it back to the liver. Because researchers conclude that HDL is a scavenger of cholesterol whereas LDL carries cholesterol to the tissue, including arterial walls where it may be deposited, HDL is considered the "good guy" and LDL the "bad guy." The reality is, the body produces most of the needed cholesterol it uses, roughly 1.5 grams per day, if the body is provided enough macronutrients (protein, carbohydrates, fats, etc.). The conversion the liver does from cholesterol to bile aides in the intestinal absorption of fats as well as vitamins A, D, E & K (fat-soluble vitamins). Cholesterol also acts as an antioxidant and has anti-inflammatory properties. It improves cell signaling in support of T-cell, B-cell and other immune functions.

High cholesterol levels are attributed to longevity, as they are precursors to hormones. Cholesterol provides insulation for more efficient conduction of nerve impulses. It was reported in 1994 that elderly people who died and had high cholesterol levels died half as often from a heart attack as did the elderly with a low cholesterol (Dahl, 1992). Plaque buildup in the arteries (atherosclerosis) is not caused by fatty foods. Oxidized cholesterol, called oxysterols, is what initiates arterial plaque formation, clotting, and promotes accumulation of calcium in other areas of the body causing conditions such as sclerosis. It doesn't make sense to blame such a life sustaining molecule for cardiovascular disease.

Otherwise, good cholesterol (whether it be HDL or LDL) turns to oxysterols inside us when it is exposed to oxygen and free radical promoters, such as iron, chlorine and other chemicals and by being near electromagnetic fields. So, you see, it is not the molecule (cholesterol) that is the problem, it is an imbalance within the system allowing for the damaged molecule to be formed. You can't eliminate something the body makes but you can facilitate a healthy environment for the body to more easily maintain homeostasis.

Many processed foods containing cholesterol, processed at high temperatures in the presence of oxygen, contain what is called "trans fats" (even when they say their product is free of it!). This happens because high temperatures cause rancidity of oils. It's not the adding of trans fatty acids into their product, it's the processing. The most common are powdered egg yolks, powdered milk and buttermilk which are used in hundreds of packaged foods, including bakery goods, boxed cake and pastry mixes, pies, powdered salad dressing mixes and dried soups. Therefore, I

> You can't eliminate something the body makes but you can facilitate a healthy environment for the body to more easily maintain homeostasis.

refer to the above listed foodstuff as dead, packaged, prepared or fake (DPPF) – because they only causes imbalances in your body!

Facts Pertaining to Cholesterol

1. The more dietary cholesterol consumed, the more the body produces. This just goes to show you that the body has a mechanism of balance, or homeostasis. All we must do is provide it a balanced array of wholesome foods and be sure we are digesting well.
2. Major cholesterol-producing areas in the body include the liver, adrenal cortex, skin, intestines, and aorta. In the skin, one form of cholesterol is converted to vitamin D from the sunlight. Other forms of cholesterol are converted to steroids, hormones, and cell membrane components. *Dietary restriction of cholesterol is not wise!*
3. Cholesterol should be considered a necessary substance; your body does! It recycles about 50% of the cholesterol from bile fluids going through the small intestines. Diet contributes only 15% of total body cholesterol; 85% is manufactured by the body itself.
4. Mental illness can be contributed, in part, by low cholesterol levels. Total Cholesterol levels below 200 lead to emotional instability, low self-control, aggression, violence, & suicide (Oxford Professor David Horrobin).
5. When you deprive yourself of cholesterol and over-eat carbohydrates, the liver is forced to store carbs as sugar, where the liver converts them into cholesterol and triglycerides (these are lipids formed from fatty acids and an alcohol). Triglycerides are often elevated in obese people and among those who consume excess refined sugars such as white sugar, fructose and alcohol.

What are considered normal, healthy total blood cholesterol levels?

Although mainstream medicine currently considers 190 and above "high cholesterol," functional cholesterol levels between 200-240 mg/dl are ideal. Even higher numbers in older women are considered desirable in that they are associated with promoting longevity. LDL is the way cholesterol is transported to steroidogenic tissues, such as the adrenal cortex and corpus luteum, a process which results in the manufacturing of the anti-aging steroid, pregnenolone (the precursor of progesterone and DHEA). These steroids are called anti-aging because they are required to prevent chronic degenerative diseases such as heart disease, cancer, obesity, senility and so on (Dahl, 1992). Do I have you wondering how to get your body to convert this amazing molecule into an anti-aging powerhouse of steroids rather than into arterial plaque and calcified deposits throughout your body? Everything in proportion, or in proper balance, is good. As Dr. Lee states, "Your cholesterol level -- whether high or low -- will not be a factor in heart disease or other diseases if your thyroid functions properly and *if* your diet is healthy." (Ph.D, 2005)

Functional medicine and its science are for the purpose of bringing functionally healthy, normal ranges of blood work back into awareness. It asserts that the actual total cholesterol level alone is **not** the most important risk factor for heart disease! Alternately, its the two **ratios between the level of HDL and the total that we need to be concerned with, and secondly the triglyceride to HDL ratio.** I would add that it is not only for a cardiovascular health assessment but, just as with the balance of electrolytes, cholesterol is an important molecule for overall health. The proper ratio of the blood lipids tested for are outlined below.

Take Control

Nutrients and enzymes are lacking from your diet because you are eating processed foods, too much sugar or just poor-quality foods lacking in adequate nutrients. Another possibility of disorder is an imbalanced diet, containing too much of certain foods and not enough of others, thus the metabolic breakdown occurs.

Cholesterol Calculations

1.   Divide HDL by total cholesterol. It should be higher than 0.24

HDL/total cholesterol ratio:

- 0.24 or higher is ideal (the higher the ratio the lower risk of heart attack)
- Under 0.24 is concerning
- Less than 0.10 is very dangerous!

It is common for people with high triglycerides to have low HDL levels. These people also tend to have high levels of clotting factors in their blood, which is unhealthy in protecting from heart disease.

To determine your second ratio:

1.   Triglyceride to HDL – simply divide

- 2 or less is considered ideal (high density lipoprotein is protective against heart disease, the lower the ratio the better!)
- 4- high
- 6- much too high!

The focus has been on blood levels of cholesterol, but the real attention should be on viewing our body holistically with all the body systems working optimally. Only 10 percent of the total cholesterol is contained in the blood, the rest is in the body's tissue (throughout the body), making a blood draw merely an indication of an imbalance. The key is the management of inflammation.

As many as 76% of diabetics die from cardiovascular disease (MD, 1976). Barnes believed that the complications of diabetes are related to hypothyroidism. As you read above, sugar wreaks havoc on our system, particularly in the delicate balance in the ratio of calcium to phosphorus. Sugar depletes B vitamins and phosphorus. When phosphorus is lacking, the body attempts to maintain the optimal ratio by dumping calcium into the blood to get excreted by the avenues of elimination. When this system is inefficient, the calcium gets stored in the connective tissue (soft tissue throughout the body). Other toxins, including excess estrogen, cause soft tissue deposition of calcium. The lipids being exposed to toxins or minerals and oxygen is where the problem occurs and forms hardening of tissues.

My 2003 version of the Merck Manual of Medical Information states that the desirable total cholesterol level is less than 200 mg/dL. Less than 100 mg/dL was the "desired level" for LDL and more than 40 mg/dL for HDL. Currently, the standards are now stating that studies show those with <150 mg/dL of total cholesterol have lower rates of heart disease and stroke. Alternately, Functional Medicine has an optimal range for cholesterol at 150-220 meaning that the healthy average for total cholesterol is 185 and up to 220 is healthy. In Functional Medicine, low cholesterol is more of a concern than high.

The 2013 American Heart Association's (AHA) guidelines for statin drug treatment was recommended at the point when LDL levels were >190 (optimal levels are <130, with a range of 65-130). The new 2018 ACC/AHA Guideline on the Management of Blood Cholesterol "allows for more personalized care for patients compared to its 2013 predecessor. Among the biggest changes: more detailed risk assessments and new cholesterol-lowering drug options for people at the highest risk for cardiovascular disease" (The American College of Cardiology, n.d.). All this above statement spells are simply more ways to sell drugs. I encourage you to know your levels and specifically the ratio, utilizing all the above calculations and considering the information provided before accepting the label of having "high cholesterol." Look into the effects due to statin drugs! Did your doctor ever talk to you about lowering your LDL with food-based sterols? Sterols are similar in structure to cholesterol, also called steroid alcohols. They are a subgroup of the steroids (derived from cholesterol). Plant-based sterols work by preventing the body from absorbing cholesterol in the intestines. This in turn helps to lower blood levels of LDL cholesterol. Plant-based sterols, also called phytosterols, are found in wheat bran (Standard Process uses this gluten free portion of the wheat as part of their general supplement, Catalyn, as a source of vitamin E), sesame seeds, almonds and Brussels sprouts.

I conclude that optimal glandular wellness, thus having balanced blood sugar is foundational to all the regulatory functions that equate to our health. This is obtained from a low-glycemic diet full of high-density nutrition and the management of stress to keep the glands that secrete hormones in check.

The Breaker

Nutrient depletion causes the body's form of communication to falter. There is no doubt of the ever-growing body of evidence of our dangerously polluted environment and nutrient depleted foods. There are two things every cell of the body needs for it to survive. Those two things are adequate nerve supply and adequate blood supply. In order to thrive, the cells need the proper building blocks (nutrients). As it so happens, the quality of nutrients determines the integrity of cells. Less mutations and genetic errors occur in the replication of DNA as a normal part of regeneration when an individual is well-nourished. The danger of being nutrient deficient is that the body will absorb heavy metals in place of nutrients. It is also worthy of noting that nutrients push out toxins. So, in essence, **nutritional therapy serves to also detoxify**. Only true nutrients are recognized by the nerves and provide the oxygen-carrying capacity. I will signify the difference between what I refer to as *true nutrients* verses chemical isolates.

Vitamins are not synthesized by the body in any sufficient amount; thus, compounds are needed in small amounts from an outside source. Ideally these nutrients should be from wholesome foods and whole food concentrated supplements. The term "vitamin" is derived from the two words "vital" and "amine," amine because each component (vitamin) being discovered, was thought to have a nitrogen-containing component known as an amine. Amines associated with amino acids are vital for life.

In the late 18th and early 19th centuries, denervation and diseases led to the study of vitamin identification and isolation. If you only knew how toxic "nutritional supplements" really are, made from petroleum, coal, and synthetic chemicals; you then would understand that taking them wouldn't benefit your health, rather destroy it. There are four primary ways to determine if your supplements are made from food or synthetic chemicals. In the Supplemental Facts (found on top half of label), the vitamin will be listed as such;

Vitamin A (as beta carotene), Vitamin C (as ascorbic acid), and so on. This tells you that your vitamins are a chemical isolate rather concentrated plant source. If it does not list "(as...)" see below in the Ingredients section. Secondly, the percentage of Daily Value is an indicator. If high (in the 100's or 1,0000's of percent) it is only possible that the product is purely chemical. The third thing to look for is the ingredients and *Other Ingredients*. Here you will often see artificial flavors, food coloring etc. These are obviously toxic, even in small amounts! The fourth sign to be wary of is anything that is Trademarked. In most cases, this means the nutrient has been changed in some way to substantially alter it from its natural composition (nature's products cannot be trademarked as they are). An exception to this is the Protomophogen extracts which retain the nutrients due to their low heat, vacuum packed process.

Nikolai Lunin, a Russian surgeon, studied scurvy while at the University of Tartu in 1881. He fed one group of mice an artificial mixture of the isolated components of milk (proteins, fats, carbohydrates, and salts, as known at that time) and the other group whole milk. The mice that received only the individual constituents all died, while the mice fed normal milk developed normally. In conclusion, he decided natural foods must therefore contain small quantities of unknown substances essential to life, in addition to the above known constituents. We now know that whole unadulterated food sources of nutrition, processed raw contain the following that are referred to as cofactors:

- Co-enzymes (biotin, flavin adenine dinucleotide, lipoamide)
- Trace Elements (metallic ions Mg^{2+}, Cu^{+}, Mn^{2+})
- Precursors and activators that act as catalysts (a substance that increases the rate of a chemical reaction)
- Antioxidants (carotenoids, lutein, zeaxanthin, etc.)
- And more (known and some still unknown)

The above list of cofactors exist organically, or naturally in plants. Minerals in the form of metals (colloidal) or ending with oxide (think of these as in a rock form, very difficult to assimilate) as with many supplements, are difficult for the body to break down. Alternately, plants are designed to uptake the mineral components from the ground. When we consume the plant, we get the pre-digested, more easily assimilated, synergistic nutrients.

Synergistic is to work in synergy with each other, complementing one another. We do not have a "magnesium" or "vitamin B deficiency," but a food or enzyme deficiency! However, if the body became deficient in a nutrient, it is also deficient in all its counterparts! Therefore, supplementing with a chemical isolate does not create balance; only nature can do that. Our bodies are incredibly made but not designed to turn raw chemicals into wholesome nutrients as nature provides.

A cofactor is defined as a counter part substance to an enzyme necissary for its function. Food Enzymes (amylase, protease, lipase, sucrase, bromelain, etc) are just one group of enzymes. There are metabolic enzymes as well. The human cell contains 1300 of them and combined with cofactors, comprise up to 100,000 (enzymesciencecom) various chemicals used by our 100 trillion cells.

In my practice, for the people I see in office, I use a particular form of muscle testing (also referred to as kinesiology). When we find our answer to the faulty system, or in other words, the problem gland, deficient nutrient or what have you, the muscle becomes weak. I liken it to finding the breaker switch and flipping it back on. Kinesiology is a form of communicating with the body's nervous system. It is a remarkable body wisdom tool.

It is sensible to assume that nutrient depletion of the body results in faulty systems, thereby reasoning that simply supplementing is the correct action to take. The shortfall with this reasoning however, is that of bypassing any consideration of the basic yet primary system that governs nutritional absorption. This being the nervous system which controls the secretion of digestive enzymes beginning from saliva in the mouth all the way down the line. Peristalsis is contraction of the intestines necessary for bowel movements and this muscle contraction happens involuntarily (governed by the Autonomic Nervous System which controls the internal organs and is affected by stress). This is the short of what could be a very long and detailed description of the intricacies of the digestive system. The point being, simply thinking to take nutritional supplements is narrow minded. Taking a look at stress that, if not managed well, can wreak havoc on the nervous system. Virtually everyone I see who suffers from digestive complaints has unresolved emotional stress they are not dealing with. Holistically speaking, the best route in addressing any condition is to first look at stress and do whatever it takes to help you manage it better and at the same time nourish your body.

Is stress the root of health conditions or nutritional deficiencies? One thing I know to be true is that the two go hand in hand. It is a vicious cycle, snow-ball effect and the chicken or the egg scenario. It is said stress is accountable for 90% of all illnesses. Below is a list of what causes stress. Stress may result from a large number of factors including but not limited to the following:

Chemicals such as those that comprise cleaning agents and personal care products, fungicides, herbicides and insecticides that mimic hormones. All synthetic chemicals impair the immune system, weaken or damage the respiratory system (over time) and interfere with nutrient absorption resulting in a snowball effect of the body's reduced ability to excrete toxic waste.

Dehydration caused by lack of water intake, excessive sweating, diarrhea or drinking too much coffee or carbonated soft drinks and eating too much junk food all impair the ability of the body to absorb nutrients and oxygen on a cellular level, thereby causing stress.

Emotions (unresolved toxic emotions) have all been shown to be a major cause of stress. The different areas of emotional stress include:

- relationship stress
- low self-esteem
- depression and other psychological conditions
- emotional shock/trauma

Fungi and fungal infections, whether ingested or inhaled are harmful to all life. The byproducts of fungi are toxic to living organisms, thereby causing a myriad of complications.

Genetically altered foods are known to cause asthma, attention/concentration problems, behavioral, digestive problems, issues with the sex organs and glands and libido, memory and cognitive disorders, metabolic, perceptual and balance problems.

Heavy metals including arsenic, mercury, aluminum and lead (among others) devastate the immune system and important regulatory glands and organs our body needs to function well. These include the liver, kidneys, lymphatic system and pancreas. Heavy metals are linked to Alzheimer's and other brain diseases and learning disabilities.

Lifestyle choices in employment and/or relationships is a known source of stress.

Microwave radiation from cell phones, microwave ovens, portable radios and telephones, television sets, and other sources are known stressors with varying effects upon people for reasons currently under investigation.

Nutritional deficiencies, whether caused by poor nutrition or poor absorption of nutrients (lack of proper food digestion).

Overwork or lack of sleep

Pain - all types of pain including psychological, loss/grief, suffering from physical injury or otherwise is a cause of stress.

Pathogens such as bacteria, viruses, fungus, molds and parasites can cause stress if the body is not able to destroy and eliminate regularly. Those that had chronic bacterial infections as children are known to have a much higher risk of heart disease as adults.

Poor diet including partially hydrogenated fats, trans fats, artificial coloring, taste enhancers (MSG), artificial appetite appeasers, artificial aromatic agents, artificial sweaters, and preservatives are all harmful to the human organism, causing metabolic error therefore autoimmune diseases and cancer.

Poor immune function caused by a combination of the above cause further stress to the body and eventually creates disease.

Prescription drugs and other synthetic or toxic chemicals are never healthy or corrective to the body, thereby a source of stress.

Having multiple stressors inflict us *and* an accumulation of the above sources of stress makes it easy to see how unhealthy conditions manifest. Doing what you can to be conscious to avoid sources of stress is wise. This above list is what I refer to as *Causes of Disorder* in other forms of teachings. Rightfully so, stress and disorder can be used synonymously is this case. When the body is subjected to these various forms of stress, without correction, you can see how things go awry.

Your glands are interconnected with the nervous system which need salts (minerals) for electrical impulses to be made. Each gland requires a set of specific nutrients. For example, the thyroid requires a lot of iodine while the adrenal glands need potassium. Cells, tissues, and organs need their nutritional fuel to regenerate.

Adrenal Glands

The adrenal glands are involved in so many aspects of health. There are many repercussions of Hypoadrenia, also called adrenal fatigue. Hypoadrenia is a precursor to most all hormone imbalances. Naturally, the kidneys are affected because of the direct contact the kidneys and adrenals have to one another. Kidney dysfunction and decreased immunity are side effects of poor adrenal function. Perhaps the most common cause of adrenal fatigue (a widespread problem) is modernized living. Let's face it; when life is packed full of deadlines, appointments and irregular eating habits, as our American way proves to be, we see this health crisis in younger and younger individuals. I have witnessed even the smallest of children suffer the effects of adrenal fatigue. Infants can be predisposed to this devastating dysfunction due to the mother's status during pregnancy**. The adrenal glands are the most endangered glands due to chronic stress.**

Adrenal Stress Self Assess

- ☐ Cravings of meat, salty, and/or rich/fatty foods
- ☐ Bloated feeling
- ☐ Tiredness especially when sitting, driving, etc.
- ☐ Hard time getting up in mornings
- ☐ Poor or irregular sleeping habits
- ☐ Irritability, anger, aggressiveness
- ☐ Mood swings
- ☐ Apathy
- ☐ Depression
- ☐ Restlessness
- ☐ Hyperactivity
- ☐ Poor concentration and/or memory
- ☐ Thyroid imbalances
- ☐ Belly fat
- ☐ Bouts of rapid, pounding heart or adrenalin rush feeling
- ☐ Faintness
- ☐ Regular feeling of weakness
- ☐ Muscle and joint aches
- ☐ Allergies
- ☐ Hypoglycemia or blood sugar problems
- ☐ Excessive dental cavities

> If you have 3 or more of these symptoms you may have an adrenal hormonal imbalance. This is a self-assessment list of adrenal fatigue symptoms. There are other reasons for the above listed conditional states, and if you have more than 3 of the listed symptoms, an appointment for a professional evaluation should be made.

☐ Hair Loss
☐ Frequent feeling cold
☐ Difficulty making decisions
☐ Headaches
☐ Slow wound healing
☐ Water retention
☐ Frequent sore throats
☐ Frequent illnesses
☐ Watery, itchy eyes
☐ Excessive sweating

You may have noticed in scanning the above symptoms that many of them could easily be caused from emotional upset and those of which are left unaddressed settle into the unconscious mind. It is common then to perpetually self-perpetrate damning behaviors... so the cycle continues until you become aware of the choices paving the way and attracting reoccurring patterns. It is difficult to ascertain if the root of the issue is emotional or a physical need for nutrition that causes the imbalance in what could be affecting the endocrine system. You will see below how it is interrelated as the thyroid plays a role in utilization of calcium and also that the thyroid *is second to* the adrenals being negatively impacted.

Symptoms of low thyroid which leads to excess estrogen and low progesterone: All female problems, such as cramps (dysmenorrh) irregular, scanty or excessive menses, uterine fibroids, ovarian cysts, endometriosis, infertility, spontaneous abortion early in pregnancy (9th or 10th week), cyclic migraines, dry vagina, osteoporosis and gallbladder disease (six times higher in women than men due to excess estrogen, birth control pills), hair on face and all female cancers (ovarian, uterine, cervical).

Cabbage, kale, broccoli, cauliflower, Brussel sprouts, watercress, and peanuts all have a chemical that inhibit thyroid function when raw, so cook these foods or avoid them if hypothyroidism is an issue for you!

Awareness is always key in living out a balanced life. Try forms of introspection such as journaling (exercise examples are provided later on in this book), meditation, prayer and yoga. A particularly helpful position that induces self-awareness is called the Head to Knee pose. To do this pose, sit on the floor with your left leg straight, right leg bent heal to pelvis, knee pointing out. Exhaling reach for your feet of your outstretched leg, bowing your head (down to your knee). This rejuvenates the mind. Childs pose is also another one and both positions most people can achieve with ease. Restorative yoga's focus is to revitalize the adrenals specifically. It is more than stretching and movement as a form of exercise. Moving the body in such intentional ways has far deeper meaning and effect.

Indications of low thyroid function, referred to as hypothyroidism, includes mental, emotional and physical symptoms:

- Weakness and Fatigue
- Weight gain or increased difficulty losing weight
- Osteoporosis
- Coarse, dry hair
- Dry, rough pale skin
- Hair loss
- Cold intolerance (you can't tolerate cold temperatures, and you feel colder than others around you)
- Muscle cramps and frequent muscle aches
- Poor circulation
- Edema (water retention/swelling), in pregnancy especially; a puffy face
- Constipation
- Depression
- Irritability
- Anxiety, panic attacks
- Depression or emotional ups and downs
- Headaches
- Vision problems
- Allergies, asthma, heart disease, cancer

- Memory loss
- Insomnia
- Hyperactivity, accompanied by fatigue (hypoadrenia)
- ADD
- Abnormal menstrual cycles
- Decreased libido
- Abnormal cholesterol levels
- Decreased blood sugar, increased adrenalin and cortisol (stress hormones)
- Immune problems, chronic infections
- Cancer
- Heart disease

The Thyroid Triad

As you may have gathered, by the above list of ailments, the adrenals are a key player in your overall wellbeing as with the thyroid - a small gland, but large in affect. There isn't a tissue in the body that is not affected by the responsibilities the thyroid takes part in. You may have heard about it in relation to weight management. The health of your thyroid is much more complex than you may have thought. To sum it up, the role of the thyroid plays a critical part in the Endocrine system (fertility, weight, digestion and overall health). Furthermore, it overlaps in the function of the immune system, nutritional assimilation; specifically, calcium utilization, electrolyte balance, bone mass/integrity and joint health. This means, healthy regeneration of muscles, cartilage, bone, and healing in general.

In all reality your heart, as well as your adrenal glands are governing the function of your thyroid. I will explain briefly how this process of disorder begins. Imagine a car. In the dashboard are gauges for the battery (the brain), the pressure gauge (heart), and speedometer (adrenals). Most people assume the brain controls most of the functions, and yes it plays a big roll and so does the heart! The heart stores all the electrical impulses from the brain. So, when the heart gets tired, the brain gets called upon. When the brain gets tired, the adrenals kick in**.** The heart is the primary power source for 90% of everything the body does!

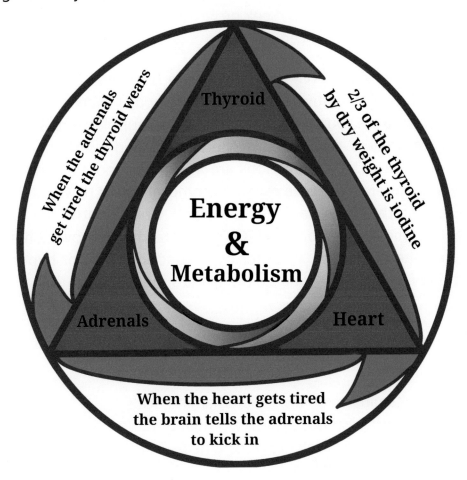

The statistics of how many in the US have a thyroid imbalance is astounding and grows larger every year. When suspected that you may have a problem relating to your thyroid, you make a doctor's appointment right? Many times, tests do not show an abnormal function and you are left perplexed with no answers and still afflicted with symptoms.

The best thing to do is to see a natural health care provider who addresses underlying thyroid issues or a functional medicine provider. In the meantime, there are simple ways to determine the function of the thyroid. Below will be some ways you can assess yourself for the need to support your thyroid. Seek professional guidance to confirm the degree of your thyroid function via advanced testing.

Containing a concentrated source of bio-available nutrients, glandular extracts are very beneficial for the regenerative capacity of the gland(s). Standard Process provides health care professionals a source of quality nutritional supplements based on Weston Price and other researchers' discoveries of the diets of, and nutritional composition of many primitive cultures. The formulations are all whole food concentrates. Standard Process is the only carrier of what are called Protomorphogens (PMG's). These glandular supplements contain the nucleic acids of the gland, which control the function of the gland. The therapeutic application of PMG's promotes healing over time. These PMG extracts regulate the glands; so, whether hypo (under-active) or hyper (overactive), supplementation of PMG's will normalize the gland's function.

Avoid These Supplements (especially if you have a glandular imbalance... *and who doesn't?***):**

1. Synthetic vitamins, minerals, isolated amino acids
2. All unsaturated oils: flaxseed oil, borage, beta-carotene, soybean, safflower, DHA, EPA, sometimes called EFA or omega-3 and-6 oils.
3. Melatonin (raises estrogen)
4. Tryptophan and 5-HTP (carcinogenic and raises serotonin)
5. St. John's Wort (raises serotonin)
6. Chelated minerals (with amino acids) – some of these are very toxic, especially glutamates and aspartates
7. Colloidal silver (just a tad less toxic than lead)

8. Colloidal minerals (most contain large amounts of toxic minerals, such as Aluminum)
9. Coral calcium (an expensive form of calcium carbonate or Tums)
10. Antacids (all of them) – a source of toxic aluminum!
11. Hydrochloric acid supplements
12. Human Growth Hormone
13. Testosterone, DHEA (both readily convert to estrogen)
14. Estrogens (natural, synthetic - Premarin, herbal estrogens (black cohosh, sage, pennyroyal, licorice); estrogenic foods (unsaturated oils, soy products); xeno-estrogens (fluoride, pesticides).

Body Talk - Signals Sent to Get Your Attention

The awareness of epigenetics is on the rise, even in the allopathic medical model. A highly regarded medical professional, Dr. Mercola speaks of us humans as beings of energy, and as such, have a bioelectromagnetic component. This means the energy of every thought or feeling produces a complex shift in the biochemical makeup of your organs or body systems. Additionally, in Dr. Mercola's article he refers to, Blair Justice, PhD, author of Who Gets Sick, stating how genes account for only 35 percent of longevity (and I would add the state of health; I personally care more for *quality of life* over length of life). *This leaves the remaining 65% to diet, exercise, stress management and other environmental factors as the chief factor in wellbeing*[1].

This is encouraging, due to it being in our hands and responsibility to choose wisely the things *we do* have control over. Stress management, nourishment and products (skin care for example) being the top three I see having the most impact. "The biofield

---

[1] https://articles.mercola.com/sites/articles/archive/2010/01/23/why-your-dna-isnt-your-destiny.aspx

is the term medical science has adopted for the intricately layered vibrational energy field that is said to surround and penetrate the physical body. For thousands of years, traditional, indigenous, pre-scientific medical systems have recognized a balanced, evenly pulsing biofield as the foundation of health and wellbeing. If this balance is disrupted, it may cause illness of some sort. There are tons of therapies that focus on the restoration of this lack of balance through such methods as acupuncture, qigong, shiatsu, meditation and yoga, in addition to Reiki" – taken from Dr. Axe article referring to studies conducted by the School of Mind-Body Medicine at Saybrook University in San Francisco and the Department of Psychology at Loyala University in New Orleans[2]. Have you ever said that you feel something in every cell of your body? Well, you are quite correct. It is physiologically true that you feel at the cellular level. A neurochemical is released with every thought, feeling, and action. Modification, conversion, or any significant long-lasting adjustment to your daily habitual ways is difficult to make a shift in because of cellular memory. However, change can be easier than previously thought! You may have heard that it takes about a month to form a habit. However, you can easily incorporate a system rooted in neuroscience combined with ancient wisdom. This is best done with a group. I offer masterclasses and group sessions and programs on this topic of reprograming or breaking old patters to form new healthier habits. These masterclasses foster a sense of community, even when the group is via the internet. Being a part of something that feels like a community leads to more success.

The notion that by examining multiple prospectives is the best way to approach a problem or understanding of something, which is what is done within groups, leads me to what is called Dunbar's Number – the respective measurement of cognitive limit that a person can maintain stable relationships. This number is still the basic unit size of armies and has been sinse the 16th century. This number averages to 150 based on Dunbar's studies. How many of us have 100-250 close relationships? Dunbar speculated that such a group would need to spend half their time on relating socially to maintain cohesion. The size of a unit was due to environmental and economic need such as Neolithic farming.

---

[2] https://draxe.com/what-is-reiki/

More intimate groups of 30-50 are favorable for endeavors other than farming and professional armies. Nevertheless, Dunbar's work has shaped evolutionary psychology, statistics and business. Robin Dunbar is currently head of the Social and Evolutionary Neuroscience Research Group in the Department of Experimental Psychology at the University of Oxford[3].

Human behavior is fascinating to me and there is one thing for sure and that is we are better together. Support groups, small groups, study groups and book clubs offer a rich experience. It helps us to grow and expand our constructs. I believe lack of prospective and creativity is the only true problem we have. So, if that's the case, why not seek a new prospective?

The electrical energetics of the body, or energy anatomy is called "Prana" in Sanskrit, "Chi" by the Chinese and "vital energy" or "life force" in English. Interestingly, Chiropractic Medicine developed by Daniel David Palmer in the 1800s, discovered similar things about the energy system of the body that the Chinese philosophers had pioneered many thousands of years before Palmer. Furthermore, Palmer had no knowledge of what the Chinese had found. These findings quantify the body's energetic pathways and when blocked, stagnation, or underflow of energy occurs in one region while overflow builds up in another. This blockage is what eventually causes disease, or malfunctioning organs.

Biochemical and bioelectric properties of the cells, simply put, are composed of ionic (or magnetic) atoms that make up the fluids inside the cell. These atoms differ in electrical charge from the fluids surrounding the cells. Like magnets in centrifugal motion, this is what makes the body electrical. Through axons (the thread like part of the nervous system), electrical impulses are carried to neurons (nerves cells) and dendrites (which receive impulses from other cells). Nerve pathways that connect neurons to one another have this electrical impulse component made possible via synapsis. Synapsis is defined as

---

[3] Robin Ian MacDonald Dunbar, Wikipedia

the junction between two nerve cells, consisting of a minute gap across which impulses pass by diffusion of a neurotransmitter[4].

Amino acids are precursors to neurotransmitters, and neurotransmitters are part of the communications network of the nervous system. Amino acids make up proteins that comprise the tissue of our bodies. Neurotransmission is what makes change difficult even when it is much wanted! In other words, you may desire to change your habits, but automation of your established habitual ways overrides your will. I offer a simple 3 step process to help you align with your truth, thus desires to make lasting change. The identification process of finding whatever it is that rings true for you is step one. To be aligned in spirit, mind and body is heaven on earth; you are then free of the constraints fear has on you.

Ask yourself, Would I like to be less reactive and rather, be more responsive with a sense of empathy? To seek understanding with compassion is likely what others would want from you. Furthermore , the compassion of self is need as well. We will explore guides and introspective exercises designed to bring balance, harmony and alignment of soul, mind and body later in this book. Staring below with education on nutrition, you can glean a new level of awareness that will naturally incite more conscientious choices in diet. Subsequently, yet just as important, is what I refer to as the "inner work" to create ease of living by *automation*. This means that information alone is ineffective for the results of change one desires. Rather, it is required that a deeper shift is made for true lasting change and it is this shift I call *"automation."* I urge you to read this book in its entirety then use it as a reference. It can be thought of as course work, a guide to a system of change. This is not merely a diet plan with added stress reduction exercises, rather what I pose is a work of art that you are instructed to create. It is a work in progress and this book is to work with the deeper levels of the human experience while making conscious choices regarding diet and lifestyle. Moreover, this book may accompany you

---

[4] Oxford dictionary

through inner journeying and unraveling beliefs that no longer serve you as you realize they are now imprisoning.

Dr. Lust (Combining Old and New: Naturopathy for the 21st Century) in the answer to the question "what is Naturopathy?": "It is a distinct school of healing, employing the beneficent agency of nature's forces, of water, air, sunlight, earthpower, electricity, magnetism, exercise, rest, proper diet, various kinds of mechanical treatment, and mental and moral science". "As none of these agents of rejuvenation can cure every disease (alone)", Dr. Lust continues on, "the Naturopath rightly employs the combination that is best adapted to each individual case".

Dr. Cordingley (Thiel) summed up Naturopathy as "the science, art, and philosophy of adjusting the framework, correcting the mental influences, and supplying the body with its needed elements. Osteopathic, chiropractic, mechano-therapy, dietetics, Christian Science and other 'single branch' systems all have their day. They all do some good and gain many adherents, but it cannot be denied that all such 'branches' have their limitations, and for that reason they will all eventually have to make room for a system that includes the best of the underlying principles of all of them- and that system is Naturopathy.

This introduction would be incomplete if it did not add the beautiful idealistic definition of Edward Earl Purinton (Thiel) "Naturopathy is the perfected Science of Human Wholeness, and it includes all agencies, methods, systems, regimes, practices and ideals of natural origin and divine sanction whereby human health may be restored, enhanced, maintained".

Allopathy, or mainstream medicine, attributes disease largely accidental, Christian Science deems it a product of diseased imagination of which sin, suffering and all forms of evil are the cause. Naturopathic philosophy asserts that disease stems from a violation of natural law. Naturopathic practices aim to tailor to the individual, not the diagnosis. Thus, poor blood as one foundational cause of disease from a Naturopathic view would then outline the course of action to find the source rather than to label (diagnose) and treat with the addition of more poisons (pharmaceuticals).

Symptoms are an expression of the body's effort made to heal itself and are not the cause of disease. Naturopathic Principles are based on six core concepts (in bold):

The healing power of nature — vis medicatrix naturae

The innate intelligence of the body to heal itself is does so through the response of the life force once underlying causes of disease have been identified (**identify and treat the cause** — tolle causam) and removed. Causes include physical, mental-emotional, social, spiritual, environmental and genetic. **Addressing the whole person** - in perturbato animo sicut in corpore sanitas esse non potest, is the responsibility of the natural practitioner. **First do no harm** — primum no nocere and **prevention** — principiis obsta: sero medicina curatur are fairly self-explanatory, and lastly, **Doctor as teacher** — docere is the principle that naturopaths are facilitators of health. We teach, guide and encourage.

Vital Nutrients, Assimilation & The Microbiome

Minerals are naturally occurring elements found in the earth. There are two groups of minerals; first is bulk minerals, which include calcium, magnesium, sodium, potassium, and phosphorus. These are needed in larger amounts than the other group, called trace minerals, which include boron, chromium, copper, germanium, iodine, iron, manganese, molybdenum, selenium, silicon, sulfur, vanadium, and zinc. Minerals are essential for every living being and to every cellular function. Minerals are needed for the formation of blood and bone, the maintenance of healthy nerve function, in the regulation of muscle tone (including the heart) and needed for the proper composition of bodily fluid. Minerals are the conveyors of electricity. They help to eliminate toxins and are catalysts which activate the functions of the body, such as the production of enzymes (both digestive and metabolic). Vitamins and amino acids cannot be utilized without minerals. Some minerals should not be taken at the same time - this can be avoided by taking angstrom sized liquid minerals which are smaller than the human cells, and therefore do not need to be digested nor do they interfere with each other's function. The liquid minerals can be customized based on your Hair Tissue Mineral Analysis if you choose to work with us professionally and utilize our laboratory services. In this form, the minerals are liquid and tasteless. Another option is whole food supplementation. Our online portal can assist you in the determination of what whole food supplements are most needed for your individuality. This is based upon the results of symptomology, easily accessed online. Your symptoms are plugged in by you into what is called a Symptom Survey then customized after a phone interview.

It is difficult to choose just three vitamins and minerals to emphasize. However, I managed to do so according to the minerals I see most often unbalanced or deficient. Everyone I've ever tested is **zinc deficient**, initially. This can sometimes be rectified by the general supplement *Catalyn*. Additionally, *Zinc Liver Chelate* may also be advised.

The most common imbalances are the ratios in calcium to magnesium, sodium to potassium, sodium to magnesium, and zinc to copper. The **ratios** between the minerals are more significant than the **levels**. This is measured by *Hair Tissue Mineral Analysis*. Please contact us for more information about the lab work. We can send you out a collection kit, which you then send directly to the lab. It isn't expensive and very much worth the information. You are provided with a booklet of recommendations and we walk you through the interpretation. Even your personalized diet is covered within the booklet. Below I will instruct you on basic dietary guidelines, but before we get to that I want to direct you to the back of this book for a guide in finding nutritional deficiencies using your nails as an indication.... Check out your body's signals of insufficient nutrition!

Zinc is acociated with normal growth and development, as it is vital for all enzamatic functions. Zinc is needed for fluid balance, heart and nervous system function, iron utilization, carbohydrate and fat metabolism. It aids in proper muscle contraction, maintains stable blood pressure and electrochemical impulses, and hormone secretion. Symptoms of deficiency include loss of taste and/or smell, high or low blood pressure, high cholesterol, chills, headaches, edema, constipation, skin problems, slow healing, indigestion, depression, nervousness, intense thirst, diminished reflux function, heart palpitations, glucose intolerance, infertility, weakness, vomiting, loss of appetite, confusion, dry skin, and protein in urine.

- Zinc is found in highest concentrations in seafood, liver, meats, fish, egg yolks, sardines, *sunflower seeds, *whole grains, green leafy vegetables, brewers yeast, and *legumes.

Magnesuim is known as the anti-stress mineral and activates nearly 100 enzymes in the body. It is needed for blood sugar regulation, enzymatic function, fat and protein metabolism, nerve and heart function, strengthens tooth enamel, reduces risk of kidney stones, heart disease, indigestion, depression, muscle cramps, and lead poisoning. Essential for cellular sodium, potassium, and calcium levels. Signs of deficiency include nervousness, confusion, irritability, depression, convulsions, skin problems, hardening of soft tissues, hypertension, arrhythmia, heart disease, atherosclerosis, blood clots, malnutrition, diarrhea, and lethargy.

- Magnesuim is in foods such artichokes, broccoli, *cashews, green beans, *navy, *black, and *pinto beans, *pumpkin seeds, organ meats, nutritional yeast, seafood, dairy, sesame seeds, spinach, swiss chard, tomatoes, and various herbs.

Potassium is important for iron utilization, fluid balance, nervous system and cardiovascular function, carbohydrate and fat metabolism, aids in proper muscle contraction, maintains stable blood pressure and electrochemical impulses, and hormone secretion.

- Highest amounts of potassium are found in tomatoes, kelp, avocado, cantaloupe, spinach, garlic, black strap molasses, peas, bananas, cabbage, spirulina, and brewers yeast

Asterisked (*) sources are those requiring special preparation in order to receive the benefit of the nutrients contained. Also note that while there may be other sources of the nutrients, I am listing only those approved sources according to the *Vital Food Plan* (my recommendations). For an example, potatoes are a good source of potassium but are not advised.

Zinc is referred to as "the missing link" for good health. There are hundreds of endogenous (produced within the body) enzymes that require an adequate level of zinc for proper function. Being a trace mineral that plays such a large roll in health and healing, a deficiency in zinc is associated with a long list of symptoms and associated with many conditions, namely skin, immune and digestive. It is vitally important that pregnant women take zinc as they are evaluated for zinc deficiency. Fortunately, there is a simple and inexpensive test for zinc deficiency that can be done quickly and easily. This test is based on a parotid salivary protein called "gustin" that is zinc dependent. Gustin is critical for the development of taste buds and olfactory sensors. The taste/reaction determines if a person has adequate tissue zinc or not. It is important for the male reproductive system as well. Zinc lost through ejaculation needs to be replaced.

Zinc works synergistically with vitamin A and is needed for the maintenance of vitamin E in the blood. It is essential for the synthesis of enzymes, hormones, collagen, insulin, and bone formation. It is also necessary for growth, regeneration, reproduction, metabolism, and wound healing. Zinc is indicated in the need for healing, alopecia, rashes and skin disorders, slow growth, low sperm count, loss of taste and smell, stretch marks, poor night vision, liver and spleen problems, loss of appetite, inflammation of the tongue, eye lid and/or mouth, infection of the nails, sickle cell disease, and Down's syndrome.

Zinc may have anti-inflammatory effects, helps to excrete toxins, regulate diabetes, reduce acne, Wilson's disease, eating disorders and weight loss. Zinc increases energy and boosts the immune system.

Fat soluble vitamins are stored in the liver, although needed daily for optimal health and regeneration (healing, growth). The below listed nutrients are what I find the most off balance in people due to over the counter supplementation or deficiency. I list "over the counter supplementation" as a cause of imbalance because these are not made from foods in proper balance. Also, hard to assimilate chemicals such as calcium citrate are used, which you may take if you would like to get kidney stones.

Vitamin A helps to form skin and mucous membranes and keep them healthy, thus increasing resistance to infections; essential for vision; promotes bones and tooth development. Vitamin A is an antioxidant that can protect against cancer. In all reality, vitamin A has many forms and is toxic in synthetic form. There is no vegetarian source of *real* vitamin A; only some 500 counterparts, the most popular being carotenoids[56] which can be converted to true vitamin A in the body, provided enough dietary fats are consumed.

5

6 Allen Tillotson, PhD The One Earth Herbal Sourcebook pg 77

Vitamin D is needed for proper bone and teeth formation and maintenance. A deficiency leads to immune problems, mental disorders, kidney and calcium absorption problems, softening of the bone (osteopenia), hair loss, skin and nail problems.

Vitamin E prevents cell damage by inhibiting the oxidation of fats and the formation of free radicals, inhibits blood clotting, retards aging, treats skin disorders, scars, wrinkles, menopause, macular degeneration, liver spots, fatigue and improves muscle strength and stamina. Vitamin E reduces blood glucose levels, risk of heart attack, prostate cancer, circulatory problems, fibrocystic breast disease, and miscarriage.

Another important nutrient is vitamin F (Essential Fatty acids or EFA's), that I simply can leave out from mentioning if I talk about vitamin D. There is a delicate balance of nutrients all needed for proper assimilation of vitamin D and calcium. Vitamin F is a key component. Therapeutic sources of EFA's include black seed currant oil, flax seeds, evening primrose oil, sesame seeds, sunflower seeds, walnuts, and wheat germ. Vitamin F supports the endocrine system (the glands which produce hormones) having a fair amount of iodine. The cardiovascular and nervous systems as well as inflammation control also rely on enough whole-food forms of fatty acids.

Consume generous amounts of olive oil (raw) and cook with coconut oil. Two tablespoons of each per day is the recommended dose. An easy to way to get in olive oil is either with salads or by adding some oil to smoothies. I like to make an herbal spice blend, sprinkle it on my salad and simply add oil and vinegar. Avoid store bought salad dressings. Even the most "natural" dressings, free of preservatives and MSG, contain polyunsaturated vegetable oils that can upset the delicate balance in inflammatory response called a prostaglandin imbalance.

Sources of Vital Nutrients

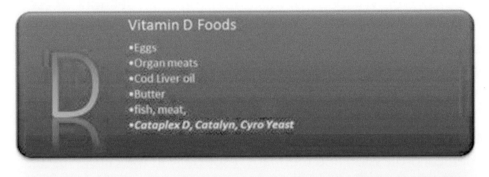

Vitamin D Foods
- Eggs
- Organ meats
- Cod Liver oil
- Butter
- fish, meat,
- *Cataplex D, Catalyn, Cyro Yeast*

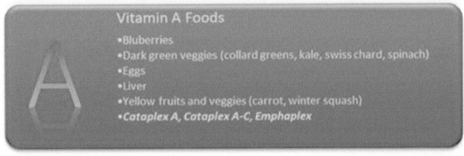

Vitamin A Foods
- Bluberries
- Dark green veggies (collard greens, kale, swiss chard, spinach)
- Eggs
- Liver
- Yellow fruits and veggies (carrot, winter squash)
- *Cataplex A, Cataplex A-C, Emphaplex*

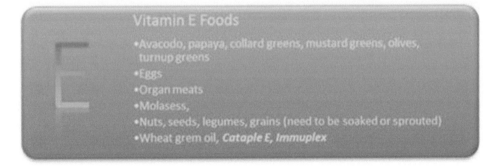

Vitamin E Foods
- Avacodo, papaya, collard greens, mustard greens, olives, turnup greens
- Eggs
- Organ meats
- Molasess,
- Nuts, seeds, legumes, grains (need to be soaked or sprouted)
- Wheat grem oil, *Cataple E, Immuplex*

Food Prep & Ratios

Like everything else, follow the money. Have you ever questioned why we can't trust the food pyramid used by dietitians and taught in our schools? Have you ever thought that perhaps it is corrupted, swayed by lobbyists that have their own agenda that benefits their pocket books? Even Wikipedia states under the grain section: *"these foods provide complex carbohydrates, which are a good source of energy but provide little nutrition."* So why then would grains consume a whopping 50-70% of the total consumption of food groups? Hmmm... regardless, I am sure by reading this, you are far more advanced in the area of dietary knowledge (enough to know about all the controversy). For fun though, I'll highlight the main issues with the food pyramid now revised by the USDA and called MyPlate as well as the most popular diets out there. Whether or not you are aware of it, to this day the medical profession and dietitians, especially in the cardiovascular department are pushing low fat as if it's the cause of heart problems. The idea that man can outsmart the maker or nature; nice try - now we have a society of diabetics (or close to) and food junkies hooked on flavor enhanced foodstuff (cereals, fruit snacks, juices, etc.) and MSG (chips, crackers and other savory convenience foods) but it wasn't intentional... it was science-based (really?). Think of all the cereal boxes on the shelves claiming "heart healthy" yet the sugar content with a non-fat milk sets you up to crave more sugar within the hour. High glucose levels equals poor heart health, chronic inflammatory conditions and degeneration. The focal point of low fats deters you away from what are considered *sacred foods* and pushes what only *sounds healthy and wholesome while instilling a fear of fat.* Has it occurred to you that the recommended 5-7 servings of fruits and vegetables, without out distinction on the wide range of nutritional qualities, could leave a gap in specificity thus lead you astray? Left to our own devices and taste buds to satisfy, it is easy to pick 5-7 sweet fruits and checkmark our standard met. Add up a berries on oatmeal, whole apple, a handful of grapes, cherries and watermelon and the amount of sugar far exceeds that which should be consumed within a day!

Sweet fruit and fruit juices were not part of the hunter-gatherer diet to the amount in which they are recommended USDA Food Pyramid. It is not often specified, what ratio of greens and non-sweet or low carb, high fiber produce to sweet fruits should be chosen. Additionally, fresh verses canned or processed in some way is lacking in the typical advice given by those who rely on their expertise.

Being at the top of the pyramid (the smallest point), it is inferred that fat should be consumed proportionally. Not only does this not coincide with healthy primitive diets but doesn't make sense with the knowledge that fats should amount to at least 30% of our caloric intake. Limiting healthy fats known to control inflammation and reduce risk of heart disease, feed the brain, required for hormone production, healthy immunity and more leaves the only other source of fats coming from dairy with its whole host of problems. The lack of differentiation of fats, i.e. saturated (as in dairy and meat), monounsaturated and polyunsaturated does not provide a good educational guide as the pyramid is intended. MyPlate, the latest version of the USDA's food guidelines, simply shows 5 categories and with further looking, does provide some tips on how to interpret the picture. The tip sheet reads: *"Limit grain, desserts and snacks, such as cakes, cookies, and pastries"* in the grains section. Furthermore, tips in the protein section list different sources of proteins to "mix up" and provide variation. It still promotes low fat yogurts and advises to choose vegetable oils over butter, as *if low fat* came from the cow! It is the fat portion in cream that contains the most vitamin A. This is why butter is deemed a healing food to those researchers of primitive diets. Why would we think that man's alterations to natural food sources would be better? Not only are we force feeding cattle grains and soy that they were never intended to consume, and I am sure that negatively affects the composition of the milk as well as the muscle meat, but the USDA promotes choosing toxic vegetable oils over wholesome fat sources! Yet, we wonder why our ever-growing population of those inflicted with chronic inflammatory diseases continue to sky rocket.

Of course, the popular keto and paleo diets must be addressed. Let's begin with the Ketogenic diet, defined as "a high-fat, low-carb diet used as a medical treatment for refractory epilepsy." This diet plan is intended to force the body into using fats as fuel rather than sugar. The brain is said to rely solely on glucose so it is unclear how the body might compensate but I believe there is risk in the long-term application of this diet. The most obvious problem is the ability to get enough fiber and greens. Supplementation can counter this if the two are administered at separate times to avoid counteracting each other. This diet requires exceptional self-discipline and commitment to upholding a nutritional supplement regimen to be successfully nourished.

Next up is the palo diet or Paleolithic (the era known as the Old Stone Age). The paleo diet is promoted as a way of improving health with the focus being on the quality of foods and also based on principles that go back to revisiting the presumed foods of long ago. It is also the time before the USDA inflicted the lobbyist groups money to promote their means of profit. This diet includes vegetables, fruits, nuts, roots, and meat and excludes dairy products, grains, sugar, legumes, processed oils, salt, alcohol, and coffee. Many people confuse the two diets or use the terms interchangeably. I'll point out here that potatoes and corn are omitted in the Paleo diet due to the health issues they pose.

Now you have a brief rundown of the two most prevalent and controversial diets being syndicated as fads. The kudos that the Palo diet gets and what sets it apart from the Atkins diet and most others is the attention to quality. It is most similar to my *Vital Food Plan*. The difference you will see is the customization opportunity of the VFP.

Protease Inhibitors, saponins and phytate, or phytic acid are discussed when you get into a deep dive of the paleo diet which is excellent to read for additional information found within this article: https://thepaleodiet.com/beans-and-legumes-are-they-paleo/

Another note-worthy diet known for healing from chronic disease is called *The Perfect Health Diet*. It too recommends traditional healing foods, and like the *Vital Food Plan*, supplements for their micronutrients including liver, kidney, egg yolks, fermented vegetables, and bone broths. Although, *The Perfect Health Diet* recommends seaweeds and shellfish which I have my concerns about so I cannot endorse them as "healing foods" as I do with bone broth, butter and egg yokes. I certainly think a quality algae supplement is good but because our ocean has become so toxic, I find it hard to imagine foods from the ocean are safe, especially because blue-green algae absorbs toxins. Algae can be sourced from companies that grow the algae in a healthy environment. Blue-green algae, cilantro and garlic taken in supplement form is a heavy metal detox protocol.

In comparison, *The Perfect Health Diet* recommends, by weight, about 3/4 plant foods, 1/4 animal foods and, as you will see in the apple shaped diagram below, beans are outlawed as part of "plant foods." By calories, *The Perfect Health Diet* aims for about 600 carb calories, primarily from starchy whole foods, around 300 protein calories and fats supply a majority (50-60%) of daily calories. I agree that more fat is needed for those in need of healing with the abundance of micronutrients, and because I am trained to test the metabolism, I know people have different needs. Individuation is what the *Vital Food Plan* allows for. Rather than pitching a standardized food plan or diet, the *Vital Food Plan* helps you evaluate your needs based on your ideal weight, constitution and multiple other factors with some basic guidelines. Most of all, you are encouraged to let your body's wisdom be the guide by being directed to pay attention and keep record of how you feel if necessary.

Yet another diet promoting the healing properties of broths as sources of fats that heal is the GAPS Diet. It is an Acronym for Gut and Psychology Syndrome. On the front of the original book are listed "Autism," "Dyslexia," "ADD," "ADHD," "Depression," Scizophrinia" and more. The developer, medical doctor Natasha Campbell-McBride formed The Cambridge Nutrition

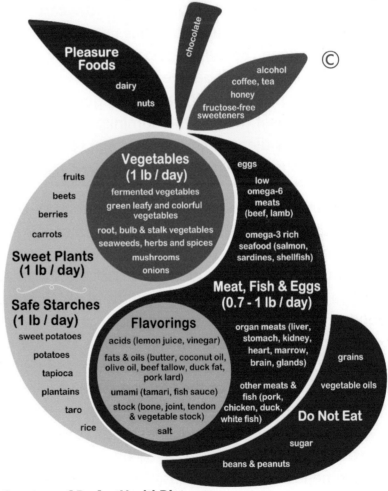

Courtesy of PerfectHealthDiet.com

Clinic in 1998. She herself had a child with learning disabilities who benefited from her protocol. I too recommended this for those in the weakest of health. There are six stages of the introduction phase of the diet. The first step is consuming solely bone broths and supplementing with essential fatty acids such as cod liver oil for a source of vitamin D and A. There is a common thread among the chronically ill and that is a severe deficiency of fat-soluble nutrients.

Of course, the popular keto and paleo diets must be addressed. Let's begin with the Ketogenic diet, defined as "a high-fat, low-carb diet used as a medical treatment for refractory epilepsy." This diet plan is intended to force the body into using fats as fuel rather than sugar. The brain is said to rely solely on glucose so it is unclear how the body might compensate but I believe there is risk in the long-term application of this diet. The most obvious problem is the ability to get enough fiber and greens. Supplementation can counter this if the two are administered at separate times to avoid counteracting each other. This diet requires exceptional self-discipline and commitment to upholding a nutritional supplement regimen to be successfully nourished.

The take-away is that keto is extreme but may be beneficial for neurological conditions. Certain other conditions benefit from a diet low in carbohydrates and this can also be accomplished with the Paleo diet without such strictness that must be adhered to as with the Ketogenic diet. I like that the Paleo diet discourages potatoes, as they seem to cause problems in many individuals. Additionally, the Paleo diet educated on legumes and the toxins if eaten without properly preparing them. Many people forget, or altogether just don't know that peanut and soy are legumes and some of the most damaging. The Perfect Food Diet discourages beans, which I believe should be kept to a minimum as with all of the legume family. I consider "safe starches" to be white rice, sweet potatoes and other root vegetables such as beets and carrots. Later on, you are given the carbohydrate guidelines within the *Vital Food Plan* and how to customize it for your needs. For example, if you have digestive complains or any medical condition, I recommend white rice because the bran of brown rice contains the bulk of the toxins that are irritating to the gastrointestinal tract. The paleodiet.com article cited above states "Starting in the early 1970's a number of scientific papers reported that consumption of raw or undercooked red kidney beans caused nausea, vomiting, abdominal pain, severe diarrhea, muscle weakness and even inflammation of the heart. Similar symptoms were documented in horses and cattle. Further, raw kidney beans were lethally toxic to rats when fed at more than 37 % of their daily calories." I have done my own research as well, but Loren Cordain, PhD, founder of the Paleo Diet movement, has 79 references listed just on the topic of legumes. So, I don't feel the need to list my own additional sources. Cordain has done great job educating the public.

4 Pillars of *HEALTHY* Food Preparation:

1. Meat on bone
   a. Be careful to not overcook it
   b. Use Moisture, time, and parts
   c. Use fat (fat soluble nutrients need fat to be assimilated)

2. Organ Meat
3. Fermentation and sprouting
4. Raw

Below is a diagram to demonstrate in quantity the portions of different food groups we should consume for an optimal diet. Details about food combining, preparations and more follows.

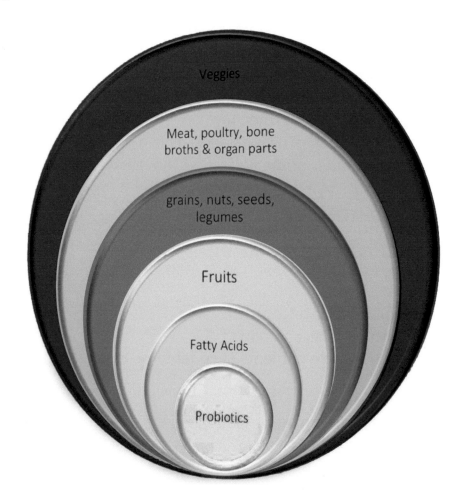

In the biggest portion, veggies are listed and defined as green leafy vegetables. Veggies should consist of a variety, as in salad greens, spinach, cabbage, kale, Swiss chard, mustard greens, etc. This should be the base to build your meal around. You may add soaked/sprouted legumes, nuts, seeds, or grains such as quinoa or millet if you are reasonably healthy with no obvious digestive issues. If you have inflammation, I recommend limiting your nuts to walnuts. These have the least amount of polyunsaturated oils that can upset the prostaglandin balance (modulating the inflammatory response). Add avocado, sprouts, mushrooms, zucchini or cucumber, bell peppers (unless you need to avoid nightshades), onions and toss with a homemade salad dressing made with olive oil. Combine with chicken or fish for an essential protein that should be eaten in small amounts. By *small amounts* I'm talking two ounces per meal and no more than four. A side dish of homemade soup makes a great addition to a well-balanced meal with plenty of nutrients. If you are wanting to lose weight, sipping on broth or a cup of soup before your salad/main course greatly reduces the appetite.

Make bone broths and vegetable stocks as the base of your soups, rice pilafs, curry dishes and more. Broths can and should consist of the glands of organically raised animals. People in need of healing inflammatory and degenerative conditions (in general and especially the gut), should consume a minimum of 8 ounces per day (by itself or in addition to meal making such as in rice pilaf).

Grains, nuts, seeds, legumes/beans need to be soaked/sprouted in order for them to be healthy. Otherwise they are ANTI-NUTRIENTS! This means consuming these foods steals from your body's reserves of nutrients in an attempt to assimilate it. These should be kept to a minimum. The short of it is that over consumption causes insulin resistance and obesity. Furthermore, it is not just the over-consumption of carbs, it is the consumption of them containing the phytic acid, saponins and other constituents that cause more harm than good by preventing the absorption of minerals. Instinctively, traditional peoples soaked or partially sprouted their nuts, seeds and grains. These foods contain enzyme inhibitors which, when neutralized by soaking or sprouting, allow for optimal digestion. Optimal digestion means that the most nutrient extraction and absorption occurs. For most nuts and seeds (including Quinoa) you'll need to soak them for 6 to 8 hours at room temperature. You can add apple cider vinegar which helps activate enzymes that neutralize the otherwise anti-nutrient factors. After soaking, drain the nuts or seeds in a colander, rinse and then dry them in a dehydrator or on the lowest setting of your oven (no more than 150 degrees).

The anti-nutrients in all grains, one being phytic acid, is present in the outer layer or bran. It adheres to minerals and can be reduced by soaking grains for minimum of 8 hours and up to 24. You can make your own sprouted grain flour by sprouting the berries, rinsing and dehydrating them and then running them through a grain grinder. Soak the raw nuts, legumes and grains in a glass container (plastic is not recommended for obvious reasons and metal pots may interfere with the process and also may leach).

By "fruits" I'm referring to sweet fruits such as berries, melons, apples, oranges, etc. - limit your amount to 1-2 servings/day. Avoid eating fruit with meals, they are meant to be consumed alone (away from all other food) so as to be digested quickly. By combining food improperly, your food literally rots, because digestion is delayed and leads to overgrowth of bad bacteria and yeast.

Fats are essential for the nervous and endocrine systems. Essential fatty acid deficiencies and imbalances are common. The easiest way to make sure you're getting enough is to add oils to smoothies, oatmeal, rice, salad dressings and to supplement with a quality fish oil. Purchase a variety of oils such as walnut, sesame seed, olive, borage, flax and evening primrose oil. Make sure to finish them within 30 days. Note that not all oils are good for everyone. Many people should avoid flax, borage, and evening primrose oils! When fat is eaten, a chemical signal is sent to your brain to slow down the movement of food out of your stomach. This is called transit time for digestion. Fat also is what causes you to feel full. Those who eat "fat-free" products tend to consume more calories than those who eat foods that have not had their fat content reduced. Fat is used not only for energy, but also for building the membrane around every single cell in your body.

Below are pointers that will guide you through the best ways to get the most nutrition through proper and complete digestion of your food. This is the first step to digestive wellness and obtaining good health in general. Also, there are many things I mention that may be good for some and not for others. This will be clarified within the following pages of this book. If you are unsure, for example about the type of oils to add to smoothies, as mentioned above, simply stick to olive oil for dressings and smoothies and coconut oil and butter for all else.

Diet is one of the most powerful tools we have that can affect every health condition. Dr. Lee said it best when he stated, "No single act or influence alters the cells of the body more than the ingestion of food." Our genetic expression is directly linked to diet, which when poor, causes more pathology and increases the intensity of signs and symptoms. If we follow what Hippocrates said and let food be thy medicine, that wisdom could be as powerful as any anti-inflammatory drug, but without the side effects! Inflammation, no doubt, causes damage. It is only wise to refrain from inflaming foods as a start to any health-improving endeavor. I'd like to remind you that any symptoms of digestive stress are a clue as to your level of inflammation. Gas and bloating shouldn't be ignored and put off until a more severe form of digestive stress or acute illness strikes. Often, people seek help from professionals when they reach a level of distress from something much more chronic or extreme, or when fatigue or not feeling like themselves causes them to miss out on life. I must point out, as minimal as gas and bloating may *seem*, it is letting us know that there is inflammation present. Even if you don't have Crohn's, colitis, celiac disease and so forth, inflammation in the gut affects us systemically. It can be the impetus of depression, headaches or insomnia and so many other conditions. Inflammation is the root of all pain and degeneration, i.e., the breakdown in the integrity of tissues. Keep in mind, the intestines share membranes with the spleen, pancreas, liver, kidneys, adrenals, bladder and female organs. This means, any prolonged issue in the gastrointestinal tract could carry over to any of the adjoining organs or glands.

Brain fog, cognitive impairment and the like may be an indication of your brain overwhelmed by the same pathological process that leads to insulin resistance and type 2 diabetes; inflammation. This growing body of research finds the link in lower levels of insulin and insulin receptors in the brain that Alzheimer's patients also exhibit. These studies make a strong argument that the over-consumption of sugars and grains, instrumental to the development of diabetes, may also result in Type 3 Diabetes (signified by "brain inflammation"). Studies show the gut, emotions and physiology/pathology are inter-related. Mindfulness based psychotherapies are now integrated into medical practices (of those healthcare providers that are interested in health, verses symptom management). I believe this interest in integration of the medical system and the mind-body link is partially due to the discovery of the gut microbiome (the name for the beneficial microbes or bacteria found throughout the digestive system). The health of one's gut is reflected in the immune system. This is an important factor when it comes to super bugs the medical establishment is faced with.

Let us first focus on proper food combining to circumvent digestive complaints and work to prevent or correct further complications caused by inflammation. Any food that is not fully digested is poisoning the body, ultimately causing inflammation and eventually subsequent disorder, or so-called disease.

There are ways to assess problems with digestion other than, or in addition to, testing for food sensitivities. Above all else, assess symptoms and dietary habits. A basic concept, yet one not surprisingly utilized in the doctor's office: The *Self-Evaluation Questionnaire* with a scoring key and recommendations is provided in the *Home Digestive Restoration Kit* (see details below).

Since the eighteenth-century blood analysis has been studied. Over three hundred years of functional medicine and nutrigenomics (including cell biology, toxicology, biochemistry, physiology, pathology, organic chemistry, microbiology and many, many more branches of the sciences) have employed technologies to unveil the molecular disorders. These immunological, neuropsychiatric, gastrointestinal and pathogenic disorders are causative factors to one's health status. These above listed branches of science, combined and applied to healthcare, are called Functional Medicine (at least in terms of my training). I combine this with the roots of original medicine in the form of Chinese and Ayurvedic medicine. I also employ methods of stress-reduction therapies as a form of healing. I believe every aspect; the mind, body and spirit, go together. However, the foundation is mindset, because without at least enough willpower to do what is necessary, all attempts fail, resulting in only more frustration, guilt, etc. I always say awareness comes first. It is key in conceptualizing, thus forming a plan for change.

Chronic stress makes chemical changes within the system which cause a wide range of symptoms. Stress, as a noun, is anything that causes strain, pressure or damage. Remember the extensive list of causes of stress above?

Whether stress be induced emotionally or caused by over-eating, the result is decreased digestive capacity. Digestion is what I would like to focus on first.

One example of stress, induced by a prolonged poor diet that leads to the removal of the gallbladder, namely constipation. The lack of bile, once stored in the gall bladder, and the lack of flow of the bile (due to the removal of the gall bladder) reduces bowel movements, causing toxicity. Because the gall bladder stores bile that emulsifies fats, intolerance in fat consumption becomes a symptom. One then avoids dietary fats, and this avoidance causes a deficiency in an important source of fat-soluble vitamin counterparts. Counterparts, or co-factors for the assimilation of some nutrients that require healthy fats leads to problems such as skin issues. If you do not have a gall bladder, you will need to forever supplement with bile salts, religiously (with every meal). Bile salts are best combined with collinsonia root to prevent the possible hemorrhoid-causing effect of bile salts, including varicose veins. Collinsonia root tones the vascular system .

Indigestion may be caused by either too much (hyperchlorohydria) or too little (hypochlorohydria) stomach acid. Many people have excess acidity, or hyperchlorohydria, caused either by the consumption of too much protein (primarily), fat and sugar, or by the ingestion of acidifying supplements such as betaine HCl and other acidifying digestive aids, and by other problems, such as acute asthma, diabetes, nephritis, and dehydration. If not caused by over consumption of the above, a mineral deficiency is the case. Either way, providing liquid minerals, the proper digestive aid enzyme formula and following proper food combining and digestive promoting ways will restore the imbalances.

Digestive enzymes are found in raw foods. They are what ripen then rot the fruit or vegetable, literally causing its decaying process and eventual demise. These enzymes in foods assist our bodies in assimilating the nutrients of the food consumed. How often do you eat raw and how old is the produce by the time it gets to your plate? The more limited in variety of foods comprised in your diet, the more depleted you likely are in digestive enzymes. In other words, the more you eat the same food that does not contain live enzymes to digest it (such as cooked and processed foods), the more the body is strained. The body manufactures some enzymes, and some are meant to be supplied in foods. It is only so long before the body is unable to keep up with the demand for the secretion of enzymes we place on it.

Over-eating is a huge cause of disease because of the burden it places on the body, especially the liver. There is no doubt that food serves as fuel for living. But what good is food if you can't digest it? In this case, it actually does more harm than good!

Food digestion is one of the most taxing, energy-consuming processes for your body. Food today, grown in depleted soils, irradiated, and processed, contains significantly less enzymes than necessary to aid in digestion. Furthermore, food cooked in health-depleting ways (fried, barbequed, boiled, roasted, pasteurized, canned, micro-waved) destroys enzymes which stresses your system greatly. A slow cooker is a good way to cook soups, bone broths, vegetables and meat without destroying the enzymes. Lacto-fermented foods such as Kim Chee are an excellent way to consume live enzymes. At health-food stores, fermented foods are readily available, or you can easily make your own! I love the Sriracha sauce that is made from Kim Chee.

Hiatal hernia, gastritis, esophageal reflux, and ulcers as a long-standing problem, usually start with fat intolerance (difficulty digesting fats and the resulting gallbladder symptoms). You may experience an array of symptoms, and certainly know of someone who is plagued with frequent burping or sour taste in the mouth, or nausea and/or pain under the right rib cage after eating, intolerance of fats or spicy foods, regurgitation of foods after meals which is worse when lying down and constipation with light colored stools. Many of these people will develop gallstones, but long before they know they have them, some of these symptoms will occur. The constant burping and the continued eating of fats and other foods that irritate the gallbladder can lead to a hiatal hernia; literally, the person burps his stomach into his esophagus. This state, if maintained over a long period of time, without the intervention of enzyme therapy and dietary changed, can progress to gastric reflux (GERD).

As you can see, good digestion is the basis of good health! Finding good food and digesting it are two separate issues. One simple test is that of your zinc status. Zinc plays a vital role in the production of enzymes   that our body manufactures. It is a common deficiency and essential for the restoration of digestion! Zinc is a trace mineral essential for healthy cell division, as well as DNA and protein synthesis, night vision, sexual maturation, fertility and reproduction, immunity, taste and appetite and so much more! There are 100 pathways that require an adequate level of zinc for proper function. The zinc test is part of the *Home Digestive Restoration Kit.*

Those with digestive issues are more likely to suffer from anxiety, depression, stress and physical ailments. This is due to the intricate relationship between the gut and the brain. You may have heard of the gut microbiome, a term describing the terrain of the gastrointestinal system relating to one's health in general.

The totality of the microbiome, including fungi, bacteria, viruses and protozoa, as molecular biologist Joshua Lederberg[7] asserts, has been heavily researched over the past decade. He states that the state of the gut microbiome effects metabolism, immune, and neuroendocrine responses. These topics span all categories of health in every area including the mind, emotional state and diseases of the brain such as dementia, schizophrenia, depression, anxiety and even personality disorders. There is a great

---

[7] https://www.sciencedirect.com/topics/medicine-and-dentistry/gut-microbiome

deal of study and continuous research being done regarding the benefits of probiotic supplementation for conditions such as psychotic disorders and autism.

Probiotic supplementation is a popular topic of late and, while I could go into great detail regarding this, rather, I encourage you to participate in our professional services to help evaluate what is needed specifically for you. There are different probiotic strands indicated for different conditions. For example, Lactobacillus reuteriis indicated for conditions of such as eczema and colic in babies whereas the probiotic Bidifobacterium longumis is specific to intestinal inflammation such as in the condition ulcerative colitis. I will, however, enumerate below some main points regarding the selection of a probiotic supplement and some misconceptions. It is of upmost importance that you seek professional assistance in choosing professional grade supplements, and probiotics are a prime example of how doing so will ultimately save you time and money.

1. More is not necessarily better. The quality and integrity of the company manufacturing the probiotic is of higher priority than the label stating a higher amount of cultures (friendly bacteria) e.g., CFUs (the culture count). In other words, convincing marketing techniques can allude to their product being "the best" because it contains a certain amount (CFUs) of probiotic strands within their product. However, this does not mean that the probiotic strands will survive the stomach acid and bile making it to the intestines where they are most needed.

2. Probiotic supplements requiring refrigeration does not automatically mean they have a longer shelf life. In fact, probiotics that do not require refrigeration are shelf stable because they do not contain live cultures that are more sensitive to temperature. Shelf stable probiotic supplements are in a dormant state and will activate in the right environment (the aim is for the cultures to set up shop in your intestines).

The bottom line is having the right strand particular to your need with the right delivery system is the most effective way to supplement with probiotics. For the best possible establishment and repair of the microbiome, it is best to include the below two different types of good bacteria.

1. Spore Probiotics or soil-based organisms (SBO) help to recondition your gut and support the growth of good bacteria; basically, they are reseeding the soil. Soil-based organisms (SBOs) are bacteria spores that work in your gut, much like the gardener. Spores provide key "reconditioning" strains of bacteria that help protect and recondition your gut flora and prepare it for the introduction of probiotics. They help your microbiome recover from on-going assaults by fluoridated and chlorinated water, stress, medications, processed foods and refined sugars, EMFs, and pollution.

2. Live probiotics are cultured foods including sauerkraut, kimchi, yogurt and beverages such as Kiefer and kombucha.

The neurotransmitter serotonin, commonly thought of as the main mood-regulating neurotransmitter, is secretory, sensory and functions in the gastrointestinal tract rather than the central nervous system. The discovery that 90% of serotonin is actually produced in the GI system led to the gut being called the "second brain."

Within the lumen of the intestine, serotonin triggers nausea and vomiting as well as altering motility which can result in diarrhea or constipation. How to heal the imbalance of this neurotransmitter? Heal the gut with Bieles Broth (recipe included in *Digestive Restoration Kit*), following the *Digestion Promoting Guidelines* and proper food combining as well as introducing pre- and pro-biotics.

Irritable bowel syndrome (IBS) is abdominal pain with alternating bowel changes from diarrhea to constipation. This can become a chronic condition of the digestive system, and also the most commonly diagnosed gastrointestinal condition. There is an enzyme formula that addresses IBS, however I must straight out of the shoot tell you the main trigger. The cause is bad fats. That's right, eliminate French fries, donuts, and bakery goods made with hydrogenated oils and other foods that sneak it in and you will improve greatly.

Malabsorption issues/nutrient deficiencies, colitis, diverticulosis, irritable bowel, constipation (un-related to hypothyroidism) ulcers, and cognitive function are related to toxic bowel syndrome. A combination of poor nutrition/nutritional deficiencies and the accumulation of toxins can lead to progressive degeneration, inflammation, and various diseases. It is imperative for a healthy immune system that all the elimination avenues (listed to the side) are in good working condition.

For many, healing means cleansing the toxic residue stored throughout the body. There are several things to remember when selecting a cleanse. Of course, it is always advisable to consult with a competent natural healthcare provider (HP) before deciding on any supplement, diet, or detoxification plan.

Below, I will list some of the considerations:

- Are you taking any pharmaceuticals that could interact with nutritionals, herbals, or any other supplement/formula?
- Are you having regular bowel movements? Talk to the professional that is assisting you in detoxing/healing to be sure they are aware of your regularity, or lack thereof. It is vital to expel the waste, so that it doesn't re-circulate and poison the body further! A good resource to look into is called the Bristol Stool Scale (also included in the kit). It is very helpful in determining abnormalities of the digestive system.
- A good health history and ideally an exam including a certain metabolic analysis can reveal some important information (kidney, liver, and glandular function, major nutritional deficiencies, etc.). Request the *Hair Tissue Mineral Analysis* Kit to test the metabolism and receive a report of explanation and recommendations. This is the best form of holistic healthcare to begin with without having to schedule a consultation.

- Are you underweight, anemic, or malnourished?
- Have you reviewed your symptoms with a healthcare provider who specializes in the areas of your concern?
- Is your body even ready to detox? If you have an inefficient thyroid or a heart problem, it may be more beneficial for your health to address those issues first. The reasoning is, certain detoxes or cleanses could over exhaust the kidneys; only worsening your problem. Again, this is assessed via the *Hair Tissue Mineral Analysis.*

An important factor in a detox protocol is the environment; if a toxic environment (home cleaning products, body care products, air fresheners or fragrance of any kind) is eliminated, the body burden is then reduced and can thus excrete much more of the buildup accumulated over the years. In my opinion, it is just as important to clean up your environment as it is to cleanse the inside of yourself. See endorsed products to help you choose chemical free household cleaning options and more HERE.

The fail-proof, safe "cleanse and repair" product (as I like to call it):

Okra Pepsin E3 – A "Gut Re-conditioner" (as stated in the *Clinical Reference Guide* provided to professionals that are authorized to distribute Standard Process products):

1. Cleanses the "sludge" off of the intestinal walls
2. Repairs damaged tissue
3. Enhances gut absorption

Indicated usages: Malabsorption issues/nutrient deficiencies, colitis, diverticulosis, irritable bowel, ulcers, constipation and cognitive function related to toxic bowel syndrome.

In comparing the use of clay and herbal preparations, I find it more effective for the purpose of detoxification, elimination, and cleansing the GI tract to gain the above three facets (cleanse, repair and enhance absorption of nutrients). In my opinion, it is far superior to cleanse the walls of the gut (re-condition) and repair the lining, thus enhancing nutrient absorption than it is to use clay and herbal concoctions. Clay is thought to promote elimination by providing "bulk" to stools by means of an insoluble fiber. It is used to absorb heavy metals and toxins, and thereby has a "cleansing" effect. There are three problems I see with this. One is the fact that a poorly hydrated or already constipated individual may become more constipated by clays. Secondly, clay will absorb the good with the bad. Essential nutrients and electrolytes are absorbed as well! This, obviously, leaves you at risk for creating deficiencies. Additionally, clay will absorb, thus decrease the action of medications and nutritional products. The benefits in light of the possible side effects/contradictions diminish the benefits of clay. I believe there are better ways to eliminate toxic metals in lieu of clay.

Okra Pepsin E3 is the multi-purpose, or double action product for healing the gut, cleansing it, or for enhancing absorption of nutrients!

Cautions:

Due to the nature of healing the gut, this product may cause seemingly "un-related changes" in mood, emotions, and cognitive function. Remember, the gut is referred to as "the second brain." And, science now knows that 90% of a "neurotransmitter" (previously thought to only be produced in the nervous system/brain), serotonin is actually produced in the gut!

General Supplements that are well tolerated any time:

- Fish oil and or 3,6,9 omega liquids
- Flax seed meal
- Goat whey (Radiant Life) – a powerful source of minerals and nutrients!

Many people may not be aware that they have less than ideal digestive function. Others rely on common tests that fail to offer the whole picture. We have discussed enzyme therapy as an option to explore and also, the detoxification quandary. After implementing the below guidelines to promote healthy digestive capacity and properly combine foods, you will glean whether or not it is necessary to seek professional guidance. The kit below is offered if you have taken all the advice within this book and still need further assistance and/or testing. Also available to you is an extensive list of symptoms relating to the organs with possible causes and a key of how to take action and prevent a hospital visit (see appendix at end of book).

Home Digestive Restoration Kit

The home kit to evaluate your digestive health includes:

1. Self-evaluation questionnaire and scoring key with recommendations based on score.
2. Stomach acidity test instructions.
3. Zinc Tally Test with an instruction sheet and the meanings of the results.
4. You will also get the recommended zinc supplement.
5. Digestive restorative essential recipe: Bielers broth handout.
6. Naturopathic Review via phone (30 minutes).
7. BONUS #1: The Unknown Physical Manifestations of Nutritional Deficiencies printout.
8. BONUS #2: a $10 off coupon towards you next purchase (or gift it to someone you care about!).

In summary, we have reviewed the basic knowledge of healthful foods and will circle back to more details within the *Vital Food Plan* later. Now I will begin with the foundational digestion promoting practices that are paramount for optimal health.

The progression of this book will build upon itself, taking you more in-depth with each layer. Implementation of the changes are feasible in stages. You will also explore

Ayurvedic wisdom in both diet and transpersonal work. As I have mentioned, healing begins within the energy body first, before it makes changes in the physical. You may wish to delve into the transpersonal content first.

Foundational Steps for Health Through Optimal Digestion

It is imperative that you follow the *Digestion Promoting Guidelines* and proper food combining outlined below. Often times this is all the change people make and they quickly receive the desired improvements.

Digestion Promoting Guidelines

- Chew, chew, and chew some more! The saliva and chewing of the food in the mouth is the first process of digestion and sends messages to the brain to tell you that you're full.
- Wait half an hour before meals, and an hour after, to drink more than 4 ounces of fluid.
- Eat fruits alone. Wait for 1-2 hours after a meal or one hour before eating. Learn more about proper food combining below.
- Always sit when eating and don't eat when feeling anxious or upset.
- Eat for nutrition not for stimulation; eat when hungry, not bored. Aim for quality not quantity of food.
- Rest comfortably after eating for at least a half an hour.
- No antacids. There are better alternatives to Tums and prescription antacids. Also, the cause must be addressed.
- Avoid meals inside three hours before bed.

More Tips:

- Take probiotics at least a half an hour before breakfast or before bed. Away from food is a more therapeutic, effective way to administer them.
- Sore throats or nausea may indicate a need to fast.
- It is best to cook with glass pots and pans; stainless steel and nonstick pans contain aluminum and when heated, especially when heating acidic and citrus foods, causes aluminum to leach into the food.
- Craving fluid while eating, bloating after a meal, itching skin, belching, gas, and difficulty digesting raw vegetables are all signs of weak digestion. Slowly build up the stomach by juicing vegetables until your stomach develops the strength to process food properly. Ask about enzyme therapy.
- Eat sprouted or soaked grains only! If you purchase them, look for gluten added in the ingredients and avoid it! Soak beans and legumes in water over night or 12 hrs. in 2T. of vinegar. Use recipes in the book *Nourishing Traditions*.

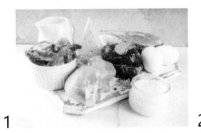 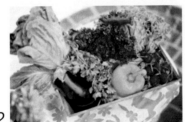 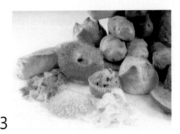

1   2   3

Proteins (picture 1) are good to combine with vegetables (picture 2) but inhibit proper digestion when combined with carbs such as in picture 3. Carbs and veggies are fine to combine.

Food Combining Summary:

Not Good to Combine:	Good to Combine:
Acid & Starch Acid & Protein Protein & Carb. Protein & Fat (as in nuts) Protein & Sugar Starch & Sugar	Protein & Veggies Starch & Veggies Starch & Fat Dairy & Fats *Always eat fruit alone! *Substitute potatoes in stew with turnips, parsnips or other root vegetables.

Food Combining 101

When combined improperly, food is not digested well. This can lead to a whole cascade of problems including candida and allergies.

1. Meat, eggs, etc. and carbohydrates need to be eaten at separate times. Protein requires more of an acidic medium for digestion (adequate hydrochloric acid in the stomach).
2. Eat meat proteins and acid foods at different times. Acid foods (tomatoes, citrus fruits) create undigested protein which putrefies, producing potent poisons.
3. Eat meat proteins and fatty foods at separate times. Some fatty foods such as nuts take hours to digest. Therefore, if taken together, neither group is digested well, and rot proliferates.
4. Eat acids and starches at separate meals. Acids counteract the alkaline medium needed for starch digestion. Again, the result is indigestion and fermentation.
5. Eat sugars (fruits) and starches separately. Fruit do not undergo digestion in the stomach and are held up with the other food causing fermentation. All fruit, especially melons, should be eaten alone.

6.   Desserts, eaten after meals, lie heavy on the stomach delaying digestion. This leads to the unwelcome fermentation of foodstuff (essentially food putrefying in the gut).

Here are some examples of how to properly combine foods for your meals:

<u>Tips</u>

More examples of ways to make meals healthy:

- Make rice with bone broth. After soaking it, cook it with the broth rather than with water.
- Easy flat bread (to replace loaves of store-bought bread). To make this simply add water to your flour of choice to make the batter the consistency you'd like. Add a dollop of yogurt or a dash of vinegar. Stir and let set 8 hours. If you do this in the morning, by dinner time it will be ready to pan fry in coconut oil. Simply add your preferred seasoning (garlic, salt, herbs) with about 1 teaspoon leavening per cup of flour used. Pour in a hot pan of oil, spread to desired thinness and cook a few minutes until golden. This is great with soups. You can substitute this for grilled cheese sandwiches by sprinkling a raw cheese on top of the hot fry bread. It is a replacement for garlic toast or can be used as a wrap to take the place of sandwich bread. Also used for breakfast or dessert with cinnamon and honey.
- Crepes are awesome options that are surprisingly easy to make. Kids love to make their own combinations. Letting children choose their toppings on pizza or fillings for crepes is a great way to get them feeling connected to their food source as well as gain a sense of control as they choose the options. Crepe combinations can include the suggestions below. Simply prepare the options and combine different combinations of fillings.
  - Pesto, bell pepper, onion

- Fresh herbs such as basil, oregano and parsley with avocado
- Artichoke, sun-dried tomato, chicken and nuts are also great additions

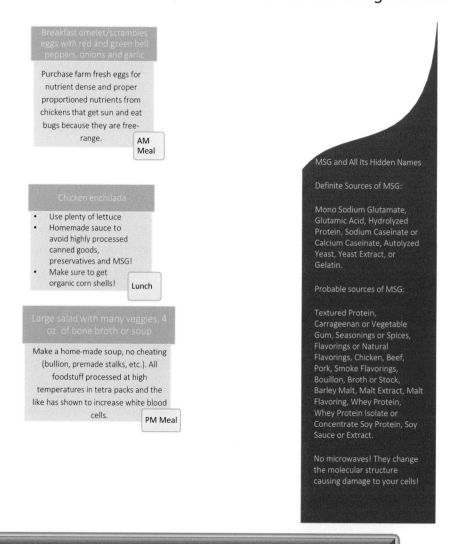

Breakfast omelet/scrambled eggs with red and green bell peppers, onions and garlic

Purchase farm fresh eggs for nutrient dense and proper proportioned nutrients from chickens that get sun and eat bugs because they are free-range.

AM Meal

Chicken enchilada

- Use plenty of lettuce
- Homemade sauce to avoid highly processed canned goods, preservatives and MSG!
- Make sure to get organic corn shells!

Lunch

Large salad with many veggies, 4 oz. of bone broth or soup

Make a home-made soup, no cheating (bullion, premade stalks, etc.). All foodstuff processed at high temperatures in tetra packs and the like has shown to increase white blood cells.

PM Meal

MSG and All Its Hidden Names

Definite Sources of MSG:

Mono Sodium Glutamate, Glutamic Acid, Hydrolyzed Protein, Sodium Caseinate or Calcium Caseinate, Autolyzed Yeast, Yeast Extract, or Gelatin.

Probable sources of MSG:

Textured Protein, Carrageenan or Vegetable Gum, Seasonings or Spices, Flavorings or Natural Flavorings, Chicken, Beef, Pork, Smoke Flavorings, Bouillon, Broth or Stock, Barley Malt, Malt Extract, Malt Flavoring, Whey Protein, Whey Protein Isolate or Concentrate Soy Protein, Soy Sauce or Extract.

No microwaves! They change the molecular structure causing damage to your cells!

If possible, shop local farmers markets to cut down on amount of chemicals, waxes, colors, and additives. Avoid irradiated food. Consume fresh produce within 3-4 days of purchase to keep food from molding and losing vitality and nutrients.

More Properly Combined Meal Ideas

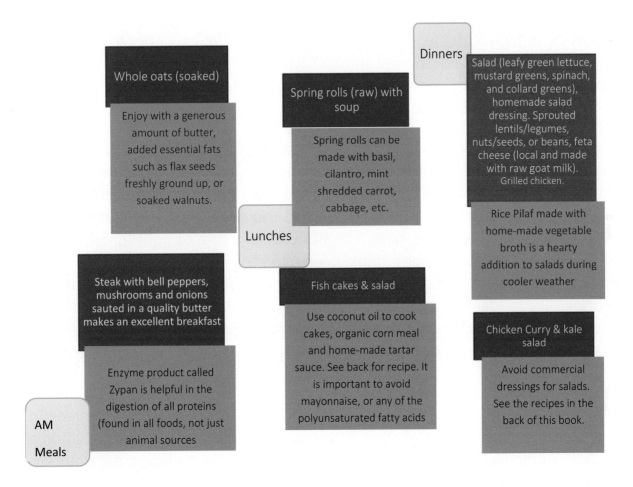

Dinners

Whole oats (soaked)

Enjoy with a generous amount of butter, added essential fats such as flax seeds freshly ground up, or soaked walnuts.

Spring rolls (raw) with soup

Spring rolls can be made with basil, cilantro, mint shredded carrot, cabbage, etc.

Salad (leafy green lettuce, mustard greens, spinach, and collard greens), homemade salad dressing. Sprouted lentils/legumes, nuts/seeds, or beans, feta cheese (local and made with raw goat milk). Grilled chicken.

Rice Pilaf made with home-made vegetable broth is a hearty addition to salads during cooler weather

Lunches

Steak with bell peppers, mushrooms and onions sauted in a quality butter makes an excellent breakfast

Fish cakes & salad

Use coconut oil to cook cakes, organic corn meal and home-made tartar sauce. See back for recipe. It is important to avoid mayonnaise, or any of the polyunsaturated fatty acids

Chicken Curry & kale salad

Avoid commercial dressings for salads. See the recipes in the back of this book.

Enzyme product called Zypan is helpful in the digestion of all proteins (found in all foods, not just animal sources

AM Meals

Step-Up Plan

You may have heard of "clean eating" and we started out this book addressing the advantages of organic and local farming. "Clean eating" is a term used to distinguish better food choices from poorer ones. If you are new to all this, there is a workup plan that may be helpful to be acquainted with.

Aim to eat healthy 80% of the time. This leaves some wiggle room for a treat or splurging on an occasion. Make deliberate choices the other 20% of the time, and don't feel guilt or give into negative self-talk. Focus on consistency and not perfection. You'll make progress and lose weight if you're making good choices often. Note: If after eating you feel sluggish, tired or lethargic, have a slight headache, sore or tight throat; write down what you ate, and any beverages drank. Keep a log to chart your reactions after eating, even subtle changes in energy levels and mood (a food log is provided at the end of this book). Try to identify sensitivities for yourself, using the record of what you have consumed with the subsequent reactions. Consider food sensitivity testing with ALCAT labs if you do not have luck with the log/charting method. You can also assess possible sensitivities to foods by pulse testing (see back of this book).

Often, beverages and unwholesome foods contain additives you may be reacting to rather than the substance itself. Also remember to follow the food combination rules, *Digestion Promoting Guidelines*. Later we will get into how to figure out your specific dietary guidelines. Furthermore, below I will detail a step-up plan for making better choices of foods.

The success in healthy and "clean" eating is for it to be intentional. Set the aim with mindset first. In other words, wrap your mind around your goal. If you intend to phase out corn for example, plan to limit it to once per week such as taco night at home with sprouted corn tortillas. If you make an intention to rotate through the meals you enjoy by making a rotation, you will be more likely to successfully reduce eating foods that you wish to limit. Below is a plan, or intentional mindset/aim in rotating through foods you may want to limit to once or twice a week only:

- Soup or a dish with lentils or beans
- A significant source of carbohydrate in the form of a sandwich or panini
- Quinoa dish
- Pasta dish
- Rice pilaf with finely chopped nuts
- Stir fry with rice

This rotation allows for you to still have the foods you are accustomed to and enjoy without the guilt of feeling like you must be so strict so as to avoid all pasta, for example, 100% of the time. Unless you need to, don't stress about being perfect and consuming only vegetables (and meat, if you are not vegetarian) rather, build in a system to allow organic options of all foods guilt free.

Soaked whole oats, rice and other grains, nuts, seeds and legumes. Sprouted seed chips and crackers. Sprouted grain bread and tortillas. Organic free-range eggs and chicken. Range-free, grass fed beef. Home ground nut butters (almond, cashew or pecan). Raw dairy. Home made dressing, dips, sauces and condiments. Omit potato chips, commercial canned goods, pasta, deli meat and fried foods when eating out.

Whole grain cereals, whole grain breads, organic chips (without "vegetable oils"), naturally flavored beverages without sugar (Zevia, Sanpellegrino). Limited canned goods, pasta, peanut butter, deli meats and dairy. Limited condiments such as mayo (polyunsaturated oils).

Read labels. Avoid MSG, GMO's, sugar and as much processed food as possible. Omit fast food. Reduce eating out. Omit "diet" foods, creamer, aspartame, energy drinks and soda. Choose real food as much as possible.

Vital Food Plan

Named for its importance, originality, and therapeutic value, the *Vital Food Plan* (VFP) is not a diet as in the commonly recognized way; as a temporary trial. Rather, the VFP is a lifestyle. It was created in combination with the nutritional experts at Nutri Spec and other researchers as well as the famous Page Clinic in Florida. The Page Clinic created a food plan based upon blood chemistry panels taken every three to four days on all patients. Dr. Page based his food plan from the early research of Dr. Weston Price and Francis Pottenger, who confirmed the relationship of the quality of foods consumed and how health was affected, both physically and emotionally. Dr. Page found certain foods to upset the body chemistry and after thousands of blood chemistry panels, Dr. Page identified foods that proved to be normalizing in the patients' blood chemistry.

Many of today's popular diets are based on the work of Dr. Page who stressed the importance in eliminating all refined carbohydrates as well as dairy completely. Dr. Page believed that it was not only important to eat quality proteins and fats, but quality carbohydrates in the form of vegetables. This food plan is designed to assist your body in its ability to create and maintain "balanced body chemistry." Make this the focus of your mentality toward your diet. There are two phases, if you choose to do a reset which includes a more strict two-week phase during which you will cut out all grains and sugar. Some people opt to also exclude dairy and animal protein and make a cleanse out of it. Depending on your individual make up, constitution and set of circumstances this may be beneficial to eliminate all of the above. However, it could be harmful to eliminate so much from your diet all at once. It is best to have an evaluation of your needs and status of health.

After the two-week reset of the first phase of the VFP (omitting all carbs) and when you are ready to re-introduce whole grains, only have them in moderation (following the amounts listed in the keys provided in the *Metabolic Regulatory Food Chart)*. If you start your day with carbohydrates, you are more likely to crave them throughout the day, and then you'll eat more and it's downhill from there so it is advised to only consume carbs in dishes such as curries and other stir-cooked dishes containing rice and soups. Absolutely stay away from breads, muffins, cookies, candies, crackers, pastas, tortillas, white rice and most baked goods. 100% rye bread is the least of the evils.

It is best to minimize grains, especially wheat. Many people are sensitive to gluten, this should be evaluated. Unprocessed rye, and a bread called pumpernickel seem to be better tolerated. Rolled oats (although not gluten free), rice, quinoa and millet can be cooked by soaking them for about eight hours with a dash of vinegar. Before cooking, replace the water with fresh water, salt and proceed to cook as normal.

Most people classify carbohydrates as either complex or simple, mainly denoting the processed grains as foodstuff such as granola and bread. Unfortunately, for most folks inflicted with digestive issues or pain, inflammation, blood sugar problems and any chronic illness, almost any carbohydrates cause dysregulation. The more you eat the more you'll want. Choose vegetables for your primary source of carbohydrates and limit grains (even the whole grains can dysregulate blood sugar). As much as I would like to promote sprouted grain breads found in stores, as of yet, I cannot find an option without added gluten. They add gluten to help the bread not crumble apart. Be sure to read the ingredients list and avoid gluten which damages the villi on walls of the intestines. Make your own or find other alternatives for bread such as home-made flat bread with soaked flour.

The problem with grains is that after harvest, the oils begin to go rancid very quickly. When scholars study disease patterns and the decline of various civilizations, many of the degenerative diseases developed when cultivation of grains became part of their culture. Allergic reactions are the result with over consumption that depletes the enzymes to digest it. This goes for any food consumed in excess. Additionally, as part of the farming practices, RoundUp™ is sprayed on many of the crops to ripen them so they can be harvested. On top of the problematic cultivation and poor soil composition, chemicals naturally found in grains such as lectins and phytic acid make them an irritant to the gut. The Paleo diet and many others are based on the finding that a handful of irritants contained in grains as well as legumes can be harmful if not properly prepared and, even then, it is advised to consume grains and legumes in minimal portions sparingly.

Across the board, it is ascertained that more green leafy vegetables are needed. Aim for as much organic, fresh (consumed within three days) and local produce as possible! It is especially important for a variety of vegetables as delineated in the *Metabolic Regulatory*

Food Chart. Make green leafy vegetables your staple including arugula, mix salad greens, spinach, chard, beet greens, kale, broccoli and mustard greens. These contain a rich deep color indicative of high nutritional content. Iceberg lettuce is one of the least nutritious types, and best avoided. Romaine lettuce however is fine. Sprouts and soaked raw nuts can be added as a substitute for croutons on salads. Don't make salads your only choice for vegetables...Get yourself and your children to consume vegetables with a tasty dip (see recipes in back of book). You can add beets to hummus, as one example.

Use olive oil and an herbal spice blend in the making of your own salad dressing. Putting together your own splash of flavor in the making of your own dressings significantly cuts down on the cost of condiments and has the added benefit of being far more healthy! Oil and vinegar blends are tasty also. You can easily make your own ranch that uses Crème Fraiche (a cultured cream made from buttermilk and heavy cream – see recipe section of this book).

The quality of your produce and the method of preparation is of upmost importance. Raw (as close to nature and un-adulterated) is preferable (depending on metabolism/ Dosha (Ayurveda Medicine)). Sauté vegetables in butter Ghee (if allergic to dairy proteins), coconut oil or true lard (be careful not to purchase so-called "lard" or "shortening" with additives). As stated in the Page Food Plan, "avoid all hydrogenated and partially hydrogenated fats – margarine and "lard" made from "vegetable oil" found in crackers, chips, bakery goods and fried foods are poison. Because peanut butter, even if raw and without the typical hydrogenation, is 28% carbohydrate, use peanuts and peanut butter sparingly."

Some metabolic imbalances are exacerbated by poly-unsaturated fatty acids primarily in the form of vegetable oils (specifically found in mayo and other condiments). While avocados, nuts and seeds contain polyunsaturated oils, they are whole foods and do not carry the same negative effects on the prostaglandin inflammatory response as do the oils extracted from these foods. You will know that you need to avoid poly-unsaturated fats if you have an inflammatory condition. Walnuts are the best choice for a source of omega 3 fatty acids if you have un-controlled inflammation.

Fats called essential fatty acids have many health-oriented people's attention for their anti-inflammatory uses and for the treatment and prevention of brain diseases and mental illness. Use generous amounts of olive oil (cold pressed, extra virgin oils can go rancid easily, add an antioxidant like vitamin E, store in cool, dark place) and coconut oil. These are all beneficial. Anyone inflicted with depression, mood disorders or mental illness, I recommend consumption of two tablespoons each of olive and coconut oils as a minimum requirement. This can help tremendously. The most suffering patients are those who have been on a low-fat diet for a prolonged time.

Fat will NOT make you fat when eaten in correct portions and within your tolerated metabolic capacity (your Dosha is to be taken into consideration here, as is the body typing). Fats are necessary in the manufacturing of hormones. Think of the danger of over-eating fat... is there any? Many traditional diets contain high amounts of fats. Current trends are promoting this once again, this is the premises of the ketogenic diet. It is far worse to become deficient in fats, thus hormone depleted, than it is to become fat deficient. There are many conditions related to not having the proper amount and ratio of fats from the diet.

Juicing is a hyped-up popular practice and, while I am not completely against it, do not advise self-administration of more than 2-4 ounces at any given time. It can however be a viable option in getting nutrients (especially for the chronically ill with impaired digestive ability as the Gerson clinic or Gerson Diet promotes). There are some cautions and concerns with juicing. Poly unsaturated fatty acids, or PUFA's are concentrated when juicing which disrupts the Essential Fatty Acid (EFA) balance in the body. This dysregulates the inflammatory response thereby many times negating one's aim. The attempted efforts to heal, reduce inflammation and correct pH via juicing results ultimately with ill effects for the long run when improperly administered. This goes for wheat grass and the "green food" products. Although it may provide an initial increase of energy for many people who are depleted in nutrients, large amounts of green foods can be irritating to your colon and should be used sparingly or in small amounts at a time. Dr. Mercola suggests not more than 4 ounces of juiced produce at a time. Flooding the system with concentrated nutrients that absorb immediately can cause upset in the metabolic regulation. While juicing does sound like a good way to bypass the digestive process for the purposes of getting the nutrients, **chewing of food is by design!** Chewing activates the part of your brain that controls your appetite and prepares your GI tract for digestion by triggering the enzyme secretion.

Juicing also often contains sweet fruits that are not advisable during the first phase and often not advisable for many with certain health issues. Once you are able to consume fruit, be careful not to do more than 1-2 servings of sweet fruits (one half apple, ½ cup berries). Fruit is pure sugar (fructose) which forms triglycerides and is ultimately converted and stored as fat. When you do eat fruit, DO NOT consume it with other foods. Remember, only eat fresh fruits alone, on an empty stomach. Eat only fresh and organic when possible. Sweet fruits, if you think about it, were not a large part of the hunter-gatherer diet (what the Paleo diet is based upon). Juice is the worst thing you can do to set off blood sugar cascade. Without the fiber in the fruit, juice sends a rapid burst of sugar into the blood stream calling insulin to the rescue. The only purpose to fruit juice is for the making of tonics such as kombucha or kefir. Water is what hydrates, no other liquid count towards hydration. In fact, coffee and alcohol require double the amount drank in water consumed plus the standard minimum requirement: calculate your need by dividing your ideal weight by 2 to get the number of ounces you need in a day. You may then divide that number by 8 to get the number of 8oz. glasses to drink per day. Good water filtration is important. Otherwise your water is de-vitalized by piping long distances and toxic by the addition of chemicals (chlorine and fluoride) as well as other environmental pollutants.

Milk is as detrimental to our health as sugar is, proclaims Dr. Page, of the Page Food Plan. Pasteurized dairy (milk, certain cheese, sour cream, half & half, ice cream, cottage cheese and yogurt) are problematic and even more so when it homogenized. The late nutritional pioneer, Arthur L. Kaslow, M.D., through thousands of his patients' food diaries, compiled a list of high-risk foods that is much the same as Dr. Page's. Dairy and wheat products were at the top of his list. The biggest problem is the alteration of protein due to pasteurization and cooking the milk as well as homogenization. Prior to homogenization of milk heart disease was virtually unheard of! Dr. Mercola does a great job educating on this topic (drmercola.com).

Raw goat and sheep milk products are better alternatives because their genetic code and fat content is apparently more like humans. Raw butter is considered the perfect source of essential nutrients, particularly vitamin A and helps with the body's utilization of fat-soluble vitamins. Butter contains what Dr. Royal Lee referred to as the "X factor," essential for healing.

There are some popular milk alternatives: soymilk, rice and nut milks. While they may sound like healthy alternatives if the aim is to avoid dairy, The Page Fundamental Food Plan asserts that "what they really are is highly processed foods that are primarily simple carbohydrates." It is easy to make oat milk and nut milks yourself. The Page Food Plan goes on to outline "Vitamite®, Mocha Mix®, and the other dairy substitutes as highly processed nutrient-depleted products that honestly should *not be* considered a food." Many of them contain dehydrated hydrogenated oils as a thickener. The alteration of oils for this purpose poses major health concerns.

Last but not least, is protein. First off, avoid soy and other highly processed foods such as deli meats, sausage and hot dogs. It is all about quality over quantity. There are twenty-two amino acids, nine of which are called essential amino acids. These are not ones that the body can manufacture, thus are essential to obtain from the diet. Amino acids are referred to as the building blocks of life because all protein is made up of amino acids that are responsible for all the functions we think of our nervous system governing. This spans from emotional responses to muscle movement. The body needs all twenty-two amino acids available so that it is not having to rob the muscles and other storehouses of amino acids. This deterioration, or breakdown, of the body's tissue can be avoided if supplied with enough of the raw materials (amino acids). Another great salad addition is to spray *Liquid Aminos* for a good salty flavor. Liquid Aminos taste much like soy sauce. Do not heat *Liquid Aminos*.

Other sources of amino acids if you are vegetarian or don't do well with animal proteins or cheese:

- Spirulina and other blue-green algae and bee pollen (to supplement with - https://www.virtualhealthcareportal.com/endorsed-products.html
- Combining soaked nuts and seeds with grains. This pairing of legumes and grains makes for a what is called a complete protein. Although I have my doubts that this alone can supply adequate amino acids, it is important to be mindful of if you are vegetarian or limit animal sources of protein.

As with the standards of the Paleo diet that has many people's attention, try to find the healthiest options available, i.e., free range and organic eggs and sources of animal meat (preferably local), whenever possible. Dr. Page says, "There is concern about pork because of its similarity to humans and an inability of pigs to sweat which results in an accumulation of toxins that is independent of their diet." Most people range from 9-12 ounces of an animal source of protein per day. This is not measured in grams because it only considered a complete protein from animal sources. Eggs are an ideal source of protein. Eat the whole egg, the lecithin in the yolk is essential for liver and brain function.

There should be some consideration to fasting, or the avoidance of animal protein which is to be evaluated on an individual basis with the help of a professional. You can calculate your personalized quantity of protein needed per day at the end of the

Metabolic Regulatory Food Chart. It is beneficial for most to consume the highest amount of protein in the afternoon. This prevents the "afternoon crash."

Amino acids may become depleted when people choose to fast. There are many amino acids that the body cannot manufacture, thus are essential to obtain from the diet. These are precursors to some fifty neurotransmitters (tiny chemicals in our body that fire signals of communication. These chemicals are what carry signals from one cell to another, also called synapsis). Knowing this highlights the fact that we need this communication, or synapsis to repair and many people that fast are seeking to heal. So, I encourage you to have an assessment before fasting.

Sweeteners: Use only a small amount of raw honey or Stevia as sweetener. Absolutely NO Nutra-Sweet, corn syrup, or table sugar. Sugar substitutes are linked to neurological disorders such as Alzheimer disease and a whole host of degenerative disorders. Although Dr. Page did not allow raw cane sugar, it does provide the nutrients (B vitamins) to aid in its metabolism. If you splurge, only raw cane sugar (called Succanat) IN SMALL AMOUNTS <2 Tablespoons in a day.

Liquids: Water is best; calculate your need by dividing your ideal weight by 2 to get the number of ounces you need in a day. You may then divide that number by 8 to get the number of 8oz. glasses to drink per day. Good water filtration is important. Otherwise your water is de-vitalized by piping long distances and toxic by the addition of chemicals and pollutants. Water is such an amazing substance. Its crystalline structure allows it to have memory and carry information. Its importance cannot be understated— there is much more to this that can be discussed. Consult with me regarding your source of water and your filtration needs. Do not alter your water's pH. If you are concerned about a pH issue, read about how to test yourself in the section in the back of this book.

Herbal teas are okay (buy bulk, most tea bags are found to have mold (trace amounts of food mold called mycotoxins. Dr. Hulda Clark talks about this danger in her book *A Cure For All Diseases*). Avoid all soda. No coffee until you are fully recovered, and then only in moderation if you have the metabolism for it. Fruit juices are forbidden because of their high fructose content and dumping of sugar into the blood stream. Broth with a meal is fine, but no more that 4oz. If you enjoy wine or beer and still insist, there are some guidelines. First, drink only with meals. Red wine has less sugar and more of the beneficial polyphenols than white wines. Most of the good foreign beer contains far more nutrients than the pasteurized chemicals called beer made by the large commercial breweries in the United States. Trader Joe's usually has a good selection. My alcohol motto: Occasional, rather than regular. Because coffee and alcohol force you to lose water, you'll have to drink more water to compensate.

Supplements: Since the fats and proteins tend to promote acid production in the body, it is very important to get enough alkalizing minerals to buffer the acid load. For this reason, vegetables are the perfect partner to small amounts of fats and animal proteins. Acidity is important in the stomach but needs to be neutralized by pancreatic enzymes and bile in the intestines. For this reason, minerals that are specific to your needs are assessed in consultations with me. Enzyme supplementation is highly recommended and my specialty (Enzyme Therapy). Screening for digestive enzyme deficiencies is one of the most important and basic evaluations you can have done and one that is foundational to health.

Regarding multi vitamin supplements, I tend to frown. All synthetic nutrients are derived from coal tar or petroleum and, in my opinion more harm than good. Feel free to ask for more information regarding the difference between the supplements I utilize in my practice and what is found on the shelves of stores.

Final Note: When uncertain, ask yourself if it is a whole food, ask your body how it feels about it, and use your best judgement. Don't consume dead, packaged, prepared or fake (DPPF). The *Vital Food Plan* is designed to help you to optimal health just as it has for the time-tested individuals that lived traditional (primitive) lives, many of whom lived into their later years without signs of degenerative diseases such as heart disease, arthritis, cancer, osteoporosis, etc. This food plan is not about eliminating foods, rather it is sound practice with the touch of intuition. You are your own best guide. Once you attain a balanced body chemistry, you will be equipped with the physical, mental and emotional regulation that your body was designed for. You will be quite pleased with the results.

Regarding the frequency of meals, some find that, smaller meals more often reduces the stress on the digestive system and increases energy level. Eating small meals can conserve energy and give your energy generator a chance to keep up with digestion by not overwhelming it when you eat a large meal. Although, this does not mean it is wise to graze. Providing the digestion, a solid two-hour break is a good idea. Frequent (every 2 hours) is recommended on occasion, per condition. For others it is best to eat three good sized meals a day – only. I recommend twice a day, called intermittent fasting, for those intending to lose weight. Again, this is one of those things that will require evaluation. The Hippocrates Institute teaches that cooked foods, with the enzymes destroyed, take up to 80% of the body's energy, adding to the body's burden while fresh raw foods only take 20% of the available energy in the processing of food. It can be reasoned then that eating frequently could pose a demand on the body that could be avoided by spacing out meals.

Insulin and other hormones are secreted in result of eating that lower the blood sugar. Often, the insulin response is too strong and within a short period of time insulin has driven the blood sugar level down. As a result of the now low blood sugar, you get a powerful craving for sugar or other carbohydrates. You then usually overeat, and the cycle of up and down, yo-yo blood sugar results. To stop this cycle, you may need more instruction and intervention as in a nutritional product to regulate blood sugar.

> Enzymes are found in all fresh foods. Enzymes are what makes them start to go bad; they literally start digesting themselves. Enzymes by definition are protein molecules found in foods.
>
> Enzyme supplementation works by assisting the breakdown process.

The most important thing to remember and strive for is consistency. Like children, adults alike thrive from it. If you prepare wholesome meals that provide the calories from quality fat, protein, and vegetables as carbohydrates, the body will function well from knowing when to expect food. Blood sugar issues will regulate with the regulation of diet. Three substantial meals are usually ideal for the majority that are trying to maintain good health. Be careful not to over-eat and follow the guidelines for promoting digestion; doing so is the single most effective self-help avenue in the wellness realm! Avoid overwhelming your body with too much to do at one time. When you sit down to eat, relax and resist the urge to multi-task. If you don't digest your food – indigestion, yeast overgrowth, gas, inflammation, food reactions, and more can result. Over-eating is a cause of disease! Americans are over-fed, yet under-nourished!

REMEMBER:

- FOODS EATEN CLOSEST TO THEIR RAW STATE OR SLOW COOKED ARE THE EASIEST TO DIGEST (for some, others benefit from cooked vegetables such as in soups). Ayurvedic evaluation assesses this, schedule a consultation if you do not know in what form to prepare your foods to create metabolic balance in yourself.
- TAKE FLUIDS MORE THAN ONE HOUR BEFORE, OR MORE THAN TWO HOURS AFTER MEALS.
- LIMIT FLUID INTAKE WITH MEALS TO < 4 OZ. BUT DRINK AT LEAST HALF YOUR BODY WEIGHT IN OUNCES PER DAY
- AVOID ICE AND VERY COLD BEVERAGES BECAUSE THEY REDUCE DIGESTIVE EFFICACY.
- NO MARGARINE, PROCESSED GRAINS OR CEREALS, WHITE FLOUR, SUGAR, FRUIT JUICES, or SUGAR SUBSTITUTES.
- CONSIDER AVOIDING the following FOODS BASED ON YOUR BLOOD TYPE

(A = dairy, mango, oranges, potatoes, tomatoes and papaya) – "A's" need to supplement with Zypan, a digestive enzyme containing hydrochloric acid (stomach acid needed for proper digestion) which is typically deficient in type A blood types.

(B = chicken, buckwheat, and peanut)

(AB = combination or all of A and B above)

(O = wheat and corn)

ADAPTED FROM THE PAGE FOOD PLAN OUTLINE

As asserted by Dr. Guy Scenker, D.C:

The following 10 dietary recommendations apply to you, your family and everyone you know:

1.   The below listed items should be avoided like the plague:

- MSG including yeast extract, and all other questionable ingredients (refer to the detailed list. I suggest you copy it and keep it with you at the time of your shopping until you learn what to avoid)
- Artificial colors
- Artificial flavors and often "natural flavors"
- All preservatives (they all contain carcinogenic chemicals and pollutants such as heavy metals)
- Anything packaged, processed and especially fast food
- Hydrogenated oils (all thickened oils) such as shortening, margarine, and foods made with them
- NutraSweet and all other artificial sweeteners (this includes gum and mints)

The above is what I refer to as dead, packaged, prepared or fake (DPPF) so common in America's diet.

2. There are 2 common dietary components that should be kept to an absolute minimum:
    -   sugar (The average person consumes over 100 pounds of sucrose every year. That constitutes an amazing 20% of their caloric intake in the form of concentrated sugar. You must understand the unavoidable health consequences of this pernicious practice. You must also understand that the sugar in fruit juice and honey is every bit as damaging as the sugar in candy.)
    -   polyunsaturated and hydrogenated oils (salad dressings, margarine, fried foods, mayonnaise). Only use olive or coconut oils, unless advised otherwise.

3. A minimum of three meals should be eaten daily (that means 21 meals each week for the average person; the elderly or those that need to lose weight may need two meals per day). Each of those meals should approximate the ideal ratio of protein and saturated fat to carbohydrate. See how to calculate your ideal carb to protein ratio within the *Metabolic Regulatory Food Chart* as well as detailed below. The ideal calculation of carbohydrates is only accomplished through our in-house metabolic testing. The point system within the *Metabolic Regulatory Food Chart* is mainly applicable only to those whom have had this testing done. However, the point system dose provide insight as to how many carb points accumulate, considering the average person is allowed roughly thirty points per meal.

4. To ensure enough protein and, especially, saturated fat intake, the following formula should be applied: Divide the body weight in pounds by 15 -- this gives the number of ounces of meat, fish, poultry or cheese a person should eat each day. (1 egg equals 1 ounce of meat.) Ideally, this quantity of protein should be divided among three meals.

To illustrate; a 120-pound woman divides her body weight by 15, which equals 8 ounces of meat, fish, poultry or cheese (or egg equivalent) daily. Dividing these 8 ounces by 3 meals gives approximately 3 ounces of meat, fish, poultry, cheese (or egg equivalent) each meal. Simple.

The proper ratio of carbohydrate to protein is achieved by calculating the carbohydrate points, which are equal to approximately 10-12 times the number of ounces of protein, depending on your metabolic needs assessed by testing (MANT). Omit this calculation of 10-12 times the amount of protein if you have not had the metabolic testing done.

Use the carbohydrate point guide within the *Metabolic Regulatory Food Chart* below. This point system eliminates counting grams of carbohydrates. For all intent and purposes, the points and carbs are interchangeable. Any foods not listed on the carbohydrate chart can be assigned the proper number of points by virtue of the food group they are in. For instance, onions are a non-starchy vegetable and therefore have the same number of points (0) as all the other non-starchy vegetables. Another example is all cooked grains; they have the same number of points as rice.

Multiply the number of ounces of protein at a meal by 10, 11 or 12 (per your test results) to arrive at the number of carbohydrate points to be consumed at that meal. An adjustment should be made in the Carbohydrate/Protein Ratio for overweight patients, and for those who are lean. For every 10 pounds a patient is overweight subtract one from the Carbohydrate/Protein Ratio. For every 5 pounds a patient is underweight add one to the Carbohydrate: Protein Ratio.

5. Find a good source of spring or well water for drinking (chlorinated and fluoridated water must be avoided).
7. As a rule, look for the least processing in your foods as possible. For example, whole grains are better than refined grains. Follow the Digestion Promoting Guidelines and Food Combining 101, listed below for proper digestion and assimilation of food.

8. Take indicated supplement(s) as a source of trace minerals and other nutrient protective factors.

9. Sunlight is a catalyst for nutrient assimilation. If you do not obtain the benefits of natural light in the eyes, health may never be regained and maintained. There are lights that emit full spectrum rays that are marketed as "mood enhancers." If suffering from SAD (seasonal affective disorder) or hormone imbalances, I would recommend the addition of this in your home, perhaps placed next to your desk/ computer to counter the effects of the artificial light source. I also recommend replacing all light bulbs with a full spectrum bulb.

Adequate sunlight can be an important part of increasing vitality. If you know of any children (or adults) with attention deficit disorder, osteoporosis, depression, anxiety or mood disorders, natural sunlight could be just the remedy! When light hits the optic nerve, an impulse is carried throughout the brain. The hypothalamus is principally where it functions as an essential regulator of hormones and autonomic nerve balance. It has been shown beyond all doubt that the depression and lethargy associated with seasonal affective disorder is nothing more than inadequate natural light and/or excess unnatural light.

10. Exercise is indispensable in promoting nutrient assimilation and utilization.

In Summary:

1. Read labels. Avoid MSG, GMO's, sugar and as much processed food as possible. Omit fast food. Reduce eating out. Omit "diet" foods, creamer, aspartame, energy drinks and soda. Choose real food as much as possible.

Whole grain cereals, whole grain breads, organic chips (without "vegetable oils"), naturally flavored beverages without sugar (Zevia, Sanpellegrino). Limited canned goods, pasta, peanut butter, deli meats and dairy. Limited condiments such as mayo (polyunsaturated oils).

Soaked whole oats, rice and other grains, nuts, seeds and legumes. Sprouted seed chips and crackers. Sprouted grain bread and tortillas. Organic free-range eggs and chicken. Range-free, grass fed beef. Home ground nut butters (almond, cashew or pecan). Raw dairy. Home made dressing, dips, sauces and condiments. Omit potato chips, commercial canned goods, pasta, deli meat and fried foods when eating out.

2. Keep the following to a minimum: sugar, refined carbohydrates, polyunsaturated and hydrogenated oils & Nutra Sweet.

3. Eat 3 meals daily, unless otherwise recommended. Sometimes during pregnancy for example, it is best to eat 4-6 smaller meals (without grazing).

4. Eat adequate animal protein and saturated fat at every meal. Avoid over-consumption of carbohydrates.

5. Drink spring or well water. Consult with us about the quality of your water and recommendations for a filter.

6. Eat animal meat cooked medium at the most (< 4 ounces per meal for most individuals). Consume vegetables according to your Ayurvedic dietary needs.

7. Eat whole, minimally processed foods.

8. Take Catalyn as a source of trace minerals and other protective factors.

9. Sunlight for your skin and your eyes is essential on a daily basis.

10. Exercise is indispensable.

If health care practitioners did nothing more than give this diet along with Catalyn, they would have achieved as much as typical "nutritionists" with their recommendations of mega dosing vitamins. Remember, the essential purposes of your diet are quite simple but are vitally important to:

1.   To ensure that you obtain adequate nutrient intake (which requires the addition of Catalyn as a source of nutrients to supplement your healthy diet).

2.   Help you achieve glycemic control — since aberrations in sugar metabolism are a causative factor in cardiovascular disease, cancer, allergies, depression and anxiety. Also, in fatigue, PMS, and in nearly every other symptom or condition you can name.

3.   To avoid highly toxic components of the common diet — most particularly vegetable oils and aspartame.

The three purposes of a diet, listed above, are the most critical dietary considerations for every person, regardless of what their symptomatic complaints may be. The solid foundation of scientific research for the truth as well as practical consideration of ancestral or natural primitive diets, should build your confidence and sense of assurance that *The Vital Food Plan* and nutritional, enzymatic and/or herbal supplements are truly the foundation in achieving and maintaining wellness. If, starting today, every woman one year prior to conceiving a child would follow the above ten above recommendations and continue following those recommendations throughout pregnancy and lactation; and, if every person followed the above recommendations from childhood through adulthood, it can easily be imagined that at least 90% of all health problems could be prevented!

ADAPTED FROM GUY SCENKER, D.C.

The last meal of the day should not be too close to bedtime. Again, it should consist of 2-4 ounces of true protein (animal source containing balanced fats and that do not convert into carbs/sugar - peanut butter being the worst) and plenty of veggies and some **soaked** legumes. Emphasis on the **soaked** because otherwise, they are anti-nutrient foods, taking more from the body than they are providing. All grains, seeds, nuts, and legumes need to be properly soaked to release native compounds in these foods which inhibit enzyme production. Be sure to not over-do on the quantity of grains and legumes. They are fillers, meaning they make you feel full and this may result in not getting enough vegetables*. Consuming an adequate amount of greens and the correct amount of everything else will provide you with the needed amount of micro (vitamins, minerals and trace elements) and macro nutrients (fat, protein, and carbohydrates/fiber).

* Consume at least one pound of greens per day. This is very important. A diet lacking in greens will make it nearly impossible to get enough calcium, iron, zinc, sodium, or selenium as well as vitamins like A, E, and K. Vegetables contain more nutrients per calorie than fruit, beans, grains, and meat. Call for your order of SP Green Food or another good fit for your supplement needs if you are not able to supply the diet with enough greens.

Fiber is a needed dietary nutrient that is typically forgotten. The average American only consumes about half the amount of fiber needed in a day. 25-40 grams/day is needed depending on being male or female. Males need more, up to 65 grams. Infant need about 13 grams of fiber, and children need 15-30. Remember that your immune system is determined by the health of your gut. Fiber is an important part of diet that contributes to immunity by supplying pre-biotics, food for pro-biotics. In other words, adequate fiber establishes a healthy environment for the good bacteria to thrive, thus establishing a healthy immune system. Good bacteria wards off the bad bacteria! There are two forms of fiber; insoluble (does not dissolve in water) and soluble, which when combined with liquid becomes gelatinous (gel-like). The herb Slippery Elm is one of my favorite fiber supplements. It is highly nutritious and a great source of soluble fiber. It's great for babies too!

Good sources of fiber include raspberries, oat or wheat bran (1oz=12grams), peas (1cup=14grams), nuts, seeds, and legumes (14-17 grams per cup).

*Fiber promotes the growth of both the good and the bad bacteria. Symptoms of dysbiosis, or an imbalance in good verses bad bacteria would consist of bloating and flatulence after consumption of high fiber foods. Apple pectin, as well as other prebiotics, would have the same effect. So, if you experience symptoms, talk with your health care provider about the need for eliminating the bad and replenishing the good gut flora. I call this the "weed and feed protocol." It entails eliminating the bad bacteria during the week and feeding probiotic supplementation on weekends. Consulting with myself or a practitioner specializing in functional medicine can guide you on testing the pathogenic composition of the gastrointestinal tract to more specifically recommend supplementation of herbs as well as probiotics.

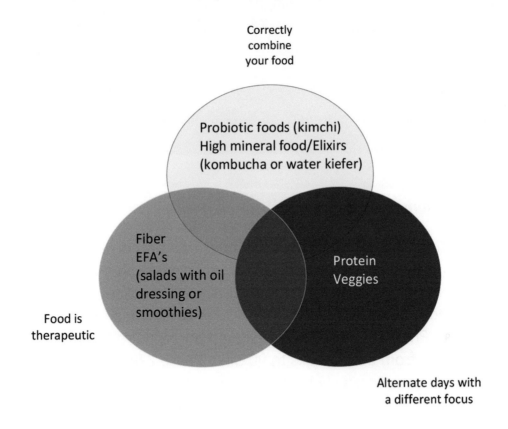

Antioxidants are natural chemicals in foods that help to fight the damaging effects of oxidation that kill cells and cause disease. Antioxidants are found in foods such as berries and other fresh fruits and vegetables. Antioxidants can also be supplements such as vitamin C and E, some amino acids and enzymes. Do not supplement with high amounts of antioxidants unless instructed to. Remember that antioxidants are only one of many identified chemicals in live or whole foods. Chemical isolates are not superior to the real deal! Your health depends greatly on a diverse and versatile diet.

Vital Food Plan Implementation

Notice on the *Metabolic Regulatory Food Chart,* the percentage columns. These categorize the amount of carbs and sugar the foods convert to. As discussed, it is not only important to eat quality proteins and fats, but quality carbohydrates as well. This food plan is designed to assist your body in its ability to create and maintain "balanced body chemistry." The Phase 1 food plan is designed for a period of time (best assessed with my help) spanning from three weeks to 90 days, Phase 2 food plan is a maintenance plan. Both can be not only extremely helpful but, in many cases, essential in controlling blood sugar and hormone imbalances while balancing many other types of biochemistry problems.

The longer you are on this food plan and the more closely you follow it, the easier it will be to maintain it. This goes back to the neuropeptides in training concept and affect.

The result in your feeling vitalized due to an improved metabolic state of homeostasis is worth the effort in establishing healthier habits. You will come to find that cravings for foods less than ideal for you will diminish. Give yourself time to change your dietary habits so you don't slip into your old way of eating. If you do find yourself slipping, I encourage you to call for an appointment as soon as possible to determine what's upsetting your biochemistry. Telecare is a new format of medicine that is becoming more utilized and certainly is effective and efficient for these purposes. Nutritional deficiencies are more prevalent than you may think and are one of the main causes of symptoms, aside from emotional dysregulation. Supplements may be needed to assist you to get back on track by reducing cravings and other symptoms.

Getting Started

Vital Food Plan 1:

The percentage you see on the charts below are the carbohydrate percentage values that tell you how much of the food converts into sugar. Learn the categorization of the foods in the chart. Fruit (sweet or sour) is not allowed for the first 90 days (Phase 1). The only exception to this is if you need natural sugar in the case of hypoglycemia or diabetes. In that case, ask for the best way for this blood sugar issue to be handled.

The 12-21% foods are not allowed at all during the initial 90 days and only occasionally after that. If you have a yeast related condition, you will want to indefinitely limit the amount of sugar converting foods along with a low or no grain and no sugar containing diet until candida free! In this case ask for the *Anti- Candida Protocol*. Those who are O blood type should stick to the phase 1 diet. Meat and veggies are ideal for O blood types with little to no fruit and always eaten alone if eaten at all.

Anyone with suspected food sensitivities does well to remain on this plan.

Vital Food Plan 2:

This is a maintenance plan. Obviously, more carbohydrates may be consumed; however, you should be evaluated before transitioning to this plan. You can self-assess if you feel confident – If not, let us help you do a proper evaluation.

For *Vital Food Plan* 2 you may experiment somewhat with how much carbohydrate tolerance your body can take. After 90 days of the phase 1 plan, your blood sugar is likely stabilized, and your metabolism set back to homeostasis. I always encourage listening to your body's signs and symptoms. Learn to crack the code; no one should know your body better! It is recommended to stay consistently as close to your calculated carb to protein ratio as possible. This ensures homeostasis.

Typically, a well-tolerated amount of fruit is a ½ cup berries (fresh or frozen, unsweetened), ½ of an apple at a time (1 apple per day), or one-inch thick slice of watermelon per day. In other words; you may have an unlimited amount of the foods in the 3% column, but not exceed one fruit from the 7-9% column. The 12-21% column is allowed in small amounts only 2-3 times per week. I recommend noting how you feel after consumption and the day after.

Elimination Diet

Some foods may be irritating your body *every time you eat them*. An elimination diet is a simple experiment that helps you to discover which foods may be causing problems (symptoms indicative of food allergies or sensitivities). The process of elimination provides the body a break from a variety of foods which calms inflammation. This is a temporary "diet". Once "trouble" foods are identified and avoided for a period of time, often once re-introduced (given the gut is healed) there are no longer reactions! If you have chronic illness, pain, inflammation, food or chemical reactions, digestive disorders or recurring health issues ask how to get started on this program successfully! *Addressing food sensitivities can be done by pulse assessment or a lab test. I recommend the Alcat test.*

Carbohydrate Limits

In Phase 1; only three servings of carbohydrates are allowed per day: The following list constitutes as one serving of carbohydrates:

- 1/2 cup white rice or pasta (cooked)
- 1 cup milk (dairy, coconut)
- 1 slice bread (any kind)
- 1/2 bagel
- 1/2 croissant
- 2 corn tortillas
- 1 flour tortilla (wrap size)
- 1/2 cup cold or hot cereal
- 1/2 cup fruit or 4 oz. fruit juice (only after 90 days or as directed AND IF candida is NOT an issue!)
- 1/2 cup popped popcorn
- 2 rice cakes – great with butter!
- 1/2 cup Rice Dream or Coconut ice cream or naturally sweetened Italian ice (not dairy)
- 6 rice crackers (or wheat (spelt, a form of wheat, is best) crackers if you're not gluten sensitive)
- 12 rice chips (or potato chips, if not night shade sensitive)
- OR ANY OF THE VEGETABLES LISTED IN THE 3rd COLUMN

Metabolic Regulatory Food Chart

The *grey italicized* color indicates foods that are off limits to the phase 1 plan and limited to the listed portions for phase 2			
3% or less carbs (consumption: unlimited)	**6% or less carbs (under 10 pts/serving)**	**7 - 9% carbs (12-20 pts/ serving)**	**OTHER**
Asparagus	***Bell Peppers**	1/cup serving:	Filtered, spring, or well water
Arugula		Acorn Squash	Bone Broths (slow cooked) – Beef, Chicken
Bamboo Shoots	Bok Choy Stems	Artichokes A, B	Caviar
Bean Sprouts	Chives	Avocado	Condiments *(ketchup, BBQ sauce, etc. made with added sugar)*
Beet Greens	Eggplant B, AB, O	Beets 12pts./cup	Dressing - Oil */ Cider or Balsamic Vinegar only*
Bok Choy Greens	Green Beans ½ cup	Brussels Sprouts	Jerky
Broccoli	Okra	Butternut Squash	The following nutrient-rich traditional
Carrot- raw	Olives A, AB, O	23pts./cup	fats have nourished healthy population
Cabbages A, AB, O	Pickles B	Carrots- cooked	groups for thousands of years:
Cauliflower A, B, AB	Pimento	10pts./cup	Butter
Celery	Rhubarb	Jicama	Beef and lamb tallow
Chard	***Tomatoes** AB, O	Leeks A, B, AB	Lard
Chicory	Water Chestnuts	**Onion**	Chicken, goose and duck fat
Chives	*Per ½ cup fresh only:*	Pumpkin A, AB, O	Coconut, palm and sesame oils
Collard Greens	*Cranberry*	Rutabagas	Cold pressed olive oil
Cucumber A, B, AB	*Grapefruit*	Sweet Potatoes 23	Cold pressed flax oil
Endive	*Kiwi A, B, AB*	pts./med. Sized B,	Marine oils
Escarole	*Kumquat*	AB, O	**_AVOID:_**
Garlic	*Pineapple*	**Winter Squashes**	The following new-fangled fats can
Kale	*Pomegranate A, O*	Yams	cause cancer, heart disease, immune
Kohlrabi		*All the below fruits are*	system dysfunction, sterility, learning
Lettuces		*between 13-30 pts per*	disabilities, growth problems and
Lemon/Lime		*½ cup:*	osteoporosis: DO NOT CONSUME
Mushrooms		*Apricot*	THESES OILS:
Mustard Greens		**Blueberries** ... *32pts*	All hydrogenated oils
Parsley		*Cherry 16pts/cup*	Soy, corn and safflower oils
Radishes		*Cantaloupe 9pts/1in.*	Cottonseed oil
Sauerkraut		*slice A, B, AB*	Canola oil
Spinach		*Guava*	All fats heated to very high
String beans		*Mango*	temperatures in processing and frying
Turnip Greens		**Nectarine**	*Sweets:*
Watercress		**Orange**	*Sugar ... ... 4pts/tsp.*
Yellow Squash		*16pts/ ½*	
Zucchini			

		Peach ... ... *25 med* *Plum* *Raspberries* ... ... *10pts./cup* **Strawberries** ... ... *12/cup* *Tangerine B, AB* *Watermelon ...* *29pts/1in. slice*	*Syrup/jelly ... ... 15 pts/T* *Alcohol* KEY THIS CHART IS ADAPTED FROM THE PAGE FOOD PLAN, WITH THE POINT SYSTEM OF THE NUTRISPEC DIET AND IN BOLD, THE EWG DIRTY DOZEN WITH LISTED FOODS CONTAINING AN ASTERISK (*) BEING NIGHTSHADES. THOSE WHO COULD BENEFIT FROM ELIMINATING NIGHTSHADE FOODS ARE THOSE WITH CHONIC INFLAMMATION AND AUTOIMMUNE CONDITIONS SUCH AS ARTHRITIS. THE BLOOD TYPE DIET IS ALSO COMBINED IN THIS CHART WITH THE LETTERS A, B, AB AND O FOLLOWING THE LISTED FOODS.
	Your ideal carb to protein ratio will be determined by your metabolic imbalances if you have been tested, your HP will have given you the ratio to strive for so you can use this chart more precisely (point system). Otherwise you may have 10-12 times the amount in carb points than in protein in ounces. For more information and examples see the expander version of the Vital Food Plan. 90 lb. IBW = 6 ounces a day or 2 ounces of protein at each of your three meals. 105 lb. IBW = 7 ounces a day or 2-2.5 ounces of protein at each of your three meals 120 lb. IBW = 8 ounces a day or 2.5 ounces of protein at each of your three meals 135 lb. IBW = 9 ounces a day or 3 ounces of protein at each or your three meals. 150 lb. IBW = 10 ounces a day or 3-3.5 ounces of protein at each of your three meals 165 lb. IBW = 11 ounces a day or 3.5+ ounces of protein at each of your three meals 180 lb. IBW = 12 ounces a day or 4 ounces of protein at each of your three meals 195 lb. IBW = 13 ounces a day or 4-4.5 ounces of protein at each of your three meals	

Each of your meals must include some protein. The easiest sources are meat, fish, poultry, or eggs. (Count 2 eggs as equal to 3 oz). Vegetarians must combine proteins carefully and consistently using a different calculation! An easy way to calculate the amount of protein you need is to divide your ideal body weight by 15 to get the number of ounces of protein to be consumed per day. This is not a "high protein diet." Like many people, you already eat this much protein during a day, but you eat it mostly in 1 or 2 meals instead of spreading it out evenly over 3 to 4 meals. If you are more physically active, eat more protein (whey powder, eggs or other animal sources containing all 22 amino acids).

Directions For Determining Your Protein to Carb Ratio:

1. To approximate the ideal ratio of protein (from animal sources) in which guarantees the balanced saturated fat to carbohydrate, ensuring sufficient protein, and especially saturated fat intake the following formula should be applied:

     a.) Divide the body weight in pounds by 15 -- this gives the number of ounces of meat, fish, poultry or cheese a person should eat each day. (2 eggs equals 3 ounces.)
     b.) Divide again by 3 for your number of ounces per meal.
     c.) Have normal serving sizes of the foods listed in columns

Different foods have been reported in different types of people having caused weight gain. I am now going to touch on body types and food choices, along with self-acceptance. There are four body types delegated and characterized by dominate glands (the thyroid, adrenals, pituitary, and the sex glands –gonadal). The book *Dr. Abravanel's Body Type Diet and Lifetime Nutrition Plan* details the chart below and provides a self-assessment questionnaire to determine your type. You can explore this avenue to further refine your dietary ideals bases upon your individual make up. To fine tune your dietary choices based on customization of your body type is yet another self-evaluation tool to explore before seeking professional guidance. You can find this assessment and the corresponding pictures of body types online to help you with this self-assessment even more.

Everyone has a body type, however, not everyone needs to follow the guidelines to a tee if not out of balance. It is, however, important to get a variety of wholesome and raw foods. A limited diet contributes to imbalance. It is necessary to follow diet plans when an apparent body type is indicated by appearance and by your metabolic typing practitioner.

Body Type Evaluation

Dominant Gland:	Cravings:	Weight Gain Area:
Gonadal type: ONLY IN WOMEN* Have a very pronounced female body, more hips than shoulders. Limit spices (they over stimulate the glands). Dill, parsley, basil, tarragon, and thyme are okay in small amounts. Limit red meat, minimum fats and oils, moderate carbs. Dairy is well tolerated. G Types do well as vegetarians. Fruit and caffeine in moderation are okay if Candida is not a problem.	Salty and Fatty Foods	Rear and Outer Thighs
Adrenal Type: Well-formed muscular and bone structure. Large Squarish head. The goal is to provide support to the thyroid and pituitary. Cut back on red meat, rich and salty foods, and cheese. Protein needs to be from fish, nuts, seeds, and legumes. Dinner can be main meal (before 6pm). Snack and all meals should consist of a complete protein. Ideal spacing of meals is 4 hours between breakfast and lunch and 6 hours between lunch and dinner.	Meat, dairy, salty, and spicy	Stomach fat- more prone to heart disease and diabetes

Thyroid type. Narrow hips, wide shoulders. Lengthy and thinner frame is the tale-tail sign of this type, thyroid types are also most common. No sweets or simple carbohydrates. There is a greater need for protein in every meal for thyroid types. Limit carbs, (and only consume whole grains) and eat lots of veggies. Rye, brown rice and millet are good. NO WHEAT. When in need of a snack have an egg or other protein but do not overcook meat. Cabbage, kale, broccoli, cauliflower, brussels sprouts, watercress, and peanuts all have a chemical that inhibit thyroid function when raw, so cook these foods if hypothyroid!

Sweets and Starchy foods

Upper Hips, Lower Tummy, and Thighs

Pituitary Type: Large skulls and a childlike appearance. Goal is to stimulate the thyroid and adrenals. No dairy, simple or refined grains, or white rice. It is best to be on a glandular or eat organ meats. Increase animal protein. Eat only when hungry but be consistent. Have a light dinner no later than 6pm.
*Basically, men are all gonadal types already...Do I really need to explain? Additionally, males can predominantly be the other three types (adrenal, thyroid, and pituitary)

Dairy
Snacking is often desired late in afternoon; you will want dairy or sweets. Try to avoid poor choices and eat nuts, seeds or animal protein.

"Baby fat allover"

Speaking of gonadal, adrenal, thyroid, and pituitary types, the supplementation of glands, called glandulars is an effective treatment for conditions of the gland i.e., hypothyroidism. Additionally, it is essential for weight loss to support these glands.

Here's how I do it...

Sundays and Wednesdays are my food prep days. I make 2 or 3 of each from the following categories. This provides the family with a variety of prepared food every three days. This means less planning, less food prep, and more free time!

Raw veggie dishes

- Carrot salad
- Raw spring rolls
- Broccoli salad
- Beet salad
- Relish tray

Veggie Dishes –Cooked

- Stir fry veggies to top rice, quinoa,
- or to make fajitas
- Soups/broths

Combo Dishes/Main Dishes

- Quinoa salad
- Curry
- Soups
- Enchiladas
- Breakfast burritos
- Breakfast sandwiches

Protein dishes *2-4 oz is all that's needed in a meal*

- Teriyaki chicken
- Roast— out of a crock pot
- Stew or soup
- Fish cakes
- Fish filet

- Boiled eggs
- Egg salad
- Deviled eggs
- Steak
- Lamb
- Chicken (limit to twice a week or less due to estrogenic effects. Chickens are fed soy)

Sugar Guidelines and Acceptable Sugar Alternatives

Ideally, I recommend that you avoid sugar as much as possible. This is especially important if you are overweight, have diabetes, high cholesterol, or high blood pressure, or any infection. Additionally, for those of us under stress or with taxed immune systems, it is also advisable to reduce and limit sugar consumption.

Weight Loss Plan

Weight loss is more than calorie restriction. It's more about the state your metabolism is in, how well food is assimilated, and how efficiently toxins are eliminated. Because of this, evaluation should be made assessing the state of metabolism (primarily the efficiency of the nervous and endocrine systems) and digestion. Your healthcare provider (HP) is your support system. Keep in good communication with your HP regarding any changes in symptoms. Supplementation should be given accordingly to help facilitate metabolic balance and better digestion of food. Diet is also tailored to your needs based on your evaluation. Below is a basic outline of the recommended daily routine to lose weight.

Cutting out sodas and sweetened beverages of all kinds is the best and easiest way of reducing sugar intake. Limiting your consumption of processed foods is not always possible at times. However, these are the most common sources of hidden sugar, so by avoiding these toxic evils found in canned and frozen foods, packaged and processed and restaurant food, you can significantly reduce your sugar consumption!

Although we do not live in ideal conditions and our lifestyle doesn't easily permit following rigid dietary guidelines, there are choices you do have control over that can help to reduce the amount of sugar in your diet.

As a standard guideline, I strongly recommend you limit your total sugar consumption to 25 grams per day and limit your fructose *from fruit* to 15 grams per day. This restriction of sugar pertains to most everyone and is especially important for those aiming to lose weight.

As a tactic to refrain from eating too much, 12-16 ounces of green tea can be consumed followed by a handful of fats, e.g. nuts. Following the *Digestion Promoting Guidelines*, consuming the tea about a half an hour away from eating is ideal. The reasoning behind eating nuts as a source of fat is because fat is what causes you to feel full. It is normal to not be satisfied after just a handful of food but wait twenty minutes and you should feel somewhat satiated. If this is repeatedly not the case, investigate pathogens as the cause. Parasites and/or candida may need to be addressed.

> *Hydrogenated oils, MSG, and other additives or preservatives are highly addictive. They increase appetite and lower immunity. These toxins build up in your body, leading to disease. Metabolic and endocrine disorders caused by poor choices in food are a cause of obesity!*

Fermented foods and beverages providing a source of probiotics is also another way to feel full. Only 4 ounces of kombucha or water kefir is needed at a time. Such beverages are a tasty treat; just watch the sugar consumption. Another thing to keep in mind is the acidity on your teeth by sipping on beverages such as coffee and cultured drinks. Rather than sipping on such beverages throughout the day, consume them all at once to preserve your tooth enamel and finish with water or by brushing your teeth.

Cultured food such as sauerkraut and kimchi can be added to salads and scrambled eggs. I notice when my teenage son has fermented foods or beverages regularly, his appetite is healthy and non-indulgent. People experience less cravings for sweets and more regulated appetites when the gut microbiome is balanced.

It is an overwhelming fact that as many as a quarter of all Americans are overweight (Dr.Oz).Americans spend over 33 billion dollars every year on weight-loss programs. Homeopathy and a diet as outlined within this book will assist in achieving a good weight. Additionally, follow the basic advice in a daily ritual. Providing the body with nutrition consistently (at first) serves to tell your body that it is being fed and there is no reason to conserve energy.

Weight Loss Ritual

Remember:

1. *Exercise is imperative for real results. The Mayo Clinic suggests striving for a minimum of 150 minutes a week of low to moderate exercise or 50 minutes a week of vigorous physical activity.*

2. *Do not consume more than 25 grams of sugar a day. Stick to Vital Food Plan's indicated carb to protein ratio for your ideal weight.*

Re-shaping your figure often times means re-shaping mindset as well! Key points to discuss and gain clarity on with your HP:

- *Does consuming fat make me fat? Not likely*
- *"Low fat"* = higher sugar to flavor.
- Choose *clean* foods
- Do a parasite cleanse

Consider the professionally guided 10 day Blood Sugar Program offered to help curb cravings and shed pounds!

1. Shortly after awakening, drink room temperature water. Run your faucet for a few minutes to flush out sediment in pipes. Never use warm tap water; either warm it over the stove or let it sit out until room temp. If on a detox, follow your given instructions. Otherwise start out your day with animal protein. Eggs, steak, or homemade soup are all good choices.
2. Two hours later take recommended supplement(s) and SP Complete smoothie.
3. Two hours later more water!
4. Two more hours later is LUNCH: Salad. If this is not satisfying and you must eat bread, have gluten free, sprouted grain bread or one tortilla **if permitted**. If Candida is an issue, it is important to follow a strict anti-Candida diet by avoiding all sources of sugar that feed the yeast, including grains. Ezekiel 4:9 English muffins are much lower in calories compared to regular bread and it takes less to feel full.
5. Mid –afternoon snack: alternate every other day; a fiber shake one day and green food supplement on day two. This allows for enough nutrition to absorb and enough fiber to detox. So essentially day one is "nutrition" day, and day two is fiber day.
6. If on a parasite detox; take the herbal tincture with water and luvos clay 15 min later.
7. Dinner should consist of salad and permitted meat, soup, a stir cooked dish with rice or quinoa (½ c. only) such as a curry dish.

8.   Two hours after dinner, drink a large glass of water and/or some tea. Store bought tea is NOT recommended (contaminated with food mold, poor quality due to irradiation. Buy bulk from Mountain Rose Herbs.com).

9.   A bowl of berries, an apple or ideally half a grapefruit. Do not use sugar to sweeten. Instead use stevia, a natural plant that can be eaten for dessert but no later than 6pm and only if Candida is not an issue nor if it interferes with any metabolic imbalance (Metabolic Type).

Juicing is a great pick-me-up if done right with only fresh veggies and no sugar filled fruits. Make sure you are juicing for your Ayurvedic Dosha or, in other words, metabolic type (we will get to that below) and using very little, if any, fruit. ONLY JUICE WITH PULP INTACT! Never juice with a standard juicer that takes out the pulp. If you do juice with juicer, you are left with an unbalanced food full of PUFA's that disrupt the endocrine system.

Fiber should never be taken with nutrients because it binds to them and excretes them the way it does heavy metals. Options:

a.   High Fiber Smoothie (make sure to have regular bowel movements - at least two times a day)

b.   A high essential fatty acid whole food smoothie powder or a green food supplement

The practice of self-love is important in general but especially so given circumstances of weight problems because you cannot expect the pounds to shed otherwise. I encourage you to do what I call the "Inner Work," or transpersonal work, outlined within this book as well as balancing of the energy centers.

Emotional Eating

Recognizing the difference between physical hunger/need vs. a craving out of boredom, nervousness or some other trigger will help you correct the bad habit. If you are an emotional eater, you are a good candidate for our inner work that you will encounter later in this book.

Calories

You can go online to calculate your BMI (Body Mass Index) and BMR (Basic Metabolic Rate) giving you your estimated fat percentage and approximate calorie intake. This recommendation is based on your height and weight. I suggest plugging in your ideal weight, or what you'd like your weight to be for the calorie recommendations if you choose to utilize this tool.

Another method is to multiply your ideal weight by 10 to configure your minimum calorie intake.

When I'm hungry,
I eat what I love.
When I'm bored,
I do something I love
When I'm lonely,
I connect with
someone I love,
When I feel SAD,
I remember I am loved.
~Michelle May

Sadly, the typical overweight American is overfed, yet undernourished. Below, I will outline the ways to pair foods together to get the most out of the nutrients in the foods.

Great meal ideas for those that need to cut down on portions. Below are some tips:

- Aim for low calorie, yet high nutritional content and foods that you are forced to eat slowly such as crepes. If you make them small, you can only make about two or three at a time. Over a 20-minute period, more time is spent preparing the meal than eating with no leftovers that are tempting to eat. Good combinations for crepes include artichoke hearts with pesto and spinach and or avocado, or simply zucchini and mushrooms sautéed with onions or bell pepper and avocado. Crepes make for simple tasty meals and without cheese, they are very low calorie.
- Adequate fat content is helpful for feeling full. On a salad, olive oil and avocado adds a hefty feel to your meal.
- Replace croutons with cheese-tons. Okay, that's not really what

AM - 1st thing in the morning make sure you are getting plenty of nutrients – follow your Eastern Medicine Metabolic Type (I find this the most beneficial– do the Ayurvedic Questionnaire below)

Some do well on light AM meal – raw salads or fresh fruit medleys

Others need warm nourishing bone/veggie broth and more of a filling meal

Snack - Fiber and oils can be taken together in between AM meal and lunch – this is a great opportunity for SP Complete containing plenty of nutrition from whole foods in a tasty powder. Add a fiber supplement and oil such as sesame, walnut, or olive.

Lunch - for some, this meal should be the largest meal. Hearty and diverse, but within the limits of The Digestion Promoting and Food Combining Guidelines, providing a solid foundation to good health. Combining warm foods such as soups, stocks, and curry dishes with salads, fresh raw spring rolls, or some crunchy carrot and celery sticks with hummus dip are some options. Remember to get **at least 2-3 ounces of protein** from a quality animal source three times throughout the day.

they are called but I like it – they are dried cheese crouton alternatives providing fat in lieu of carbs.

Fitting It All In

A mid-afternoon snack should contain a liberal amount of fat and protein. Examples are an egg, tuna eaten with celery sticks, bone and veggie broth with steak and zucchini, etc. No peanut butters! Other nut and seed butters are okay; however, nuts are essentially carbohydrates and not an ideal source of protein, nor are they complete proteins. Complete proteins have all 9 of the essential amino acids within the food itself. There are very few vegetarian sources of complete proteins. Nuts, seeds and legumes are not the best choice for people with blood sugar imbalances or those who wish to lose weight. These foods are also controversial as to their benefit to health and may be causing more harm than good. We went over this within the *Vital Food Plan*.

Smoothies (without fruit or any sugar) are a good option for a meal replacement. Quality whey protein powder can be the base along with a raw egg or two. I highly recommend *SP Complete or *SP Detox Balance. Animal sources of protein in the evening feeds the adrenal glands needed for energy, stress regulation, hormone balance, and even inflammation and blood sugar balance! Ask for smoothie recipes and do not purchase over the counter whey protein powders!

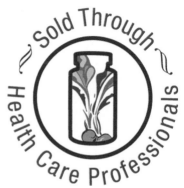

These products are only sold through healthcare professionals. If you find these accessible online, it is an un-promoted selling format. Please do not support those who choose to break the rules. Thank you.

The diagram below is a demonstration of the supplemental basic protocol everyone can benefit from.

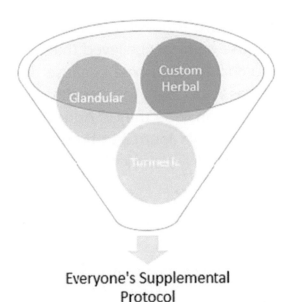

Everyone's Supplemental Protocol

A custom herbal remedy evaluated for your individual needs and constitutional make up, would be a great addition to increasing one's vitality. Additionally, turmeric in the form of Turmeric Forte has the highest efficacy of all the turmeric concoctions out there. Since the 1980's, it has been known that curcumin (a compound in turmeric) is poorly absorbed by the body (MediHerb). However, now available as a clinically tested and confirmed *Turmeric Forte's* curcumin is shown to be 24.8 times more bioavailable than equivalent products such as products that combine turmeric with other herbs or black pepper known to increase turmeric's effectiveness. Furthermore, *Turmeric Forte* was found to be 45.6 times more bioavailable than curcumins alone. This is due to the curcumin in *Turmeric Forte* being bound to fenugreek fiber. This product is formulated to down-regulate inflammation in the brain specifically. It is also effective in reduction pain in arthritis, decreased gut related issues, and allergic rhinitis (MediHerb, 2017). Clinical trials proved *Turmeric Forte* to benefit patients with cancer, kidney disease, pre-diabetes and type II diabetes, osteopenia, osteoarthritis, and more (MediHerb, 2017).

In summary, an herbal protocol, either based on your constitution or a rotation throughout the year and in alignment with the seasons. An herbal supplement is used to support your system and is a practice honored in cultures that uphold ancestral wisdom traditions. Consider booking an appointment to evaluate the longevity-promoting properties herbal medicine has to offer you in addition to *Turmeric Forte* and the pure, un-adulterated proteins of the PMG's for nutrition specifically for glandular regeneration.

Dr. Lee named his nutrition company, now called Standard Process (that partnered with MediHerb), the Therapeutic Food Company because he firmly believed that food was therapeutic. However, the FDA forced Dr. Lee to change the name because they adamantly proclaimed this not to be true – the FDA does not deem food as the same beneficial substance in the way some of us do. Even back in 1939 the US Agricultural Department's yearly journal *Food and Life* dedicated the whole Journal to how certain vitamin deficiencies have led to disease yet the powers at be set out to silence simple healthy foods. Who could this benefit?

Using our own government as a tool, the fear that was created unfortunately proved to be so prevailing and the outlandish ploy to squelch whole foods resulted in the head of the American Pharmacists Association to label Dr. Lee as a quack. This front-page article of slander in a prominent Chicago Newspaper directed towards Dr. Lee was later retracted. An apology was issued on the back page of the newspaper weeks later (Research). The initial article condemned Dr. Lee for the warning he asserted about calcium metabolism in regard to refined carbohydrates. That didn't fit in line with the American agricultural agenda.

To think that the substances you consume wouldn't have a bearing on the body and one's health is hard to comprehend. Dr. Kaslow in partnership with International Foundation for Nutrition and Health (IFNH) devoted over seventy pages just to calcium metabolism in the first chapter of the Laboratory Interpretation Desk Reference Manual. Fortunately, we have truth-seeking entities like IFNH to bring the writings of the pioneers in nutritional wellness to health-oriented practitioners. It is Dr. Lee's writings that provide us with such pivotal findings on matters of nutrition for clinical use. His knowledge upholds the foundations of biochemistry and physiology paired with the wisdom traditions, proving why and how nutrition works.

These principles have the potential to change healthcare from the disease model of Allopathic Medicine and (the pharmaceutical companies) to a model of health and prevention. Perhaps this is precisely what the industry and powers that be are afraid of.

The Road to Healing – Building Your Home Remedy Preparedness Kit

Beginning in the late 1800s homeopathic medicine became widely used in the United States. Since the development of modern medicines and ads on television that gained the hopeful hearts of many, the idea that modern medicine as the cure-all became more prominent. As this promise has largely failed our bodies' vitality, homeopathy is undergoing resurgence in our country once again. Europe and Latin America use it much more. Homeopathy is its own separate system of medicine. It was developed in Germany by Dr Samuel Hahnemann over 200 years ago. This brilliant doctor made observations and cataloged them in the materia medica. He also established the "like cures like" theory. In a homeopathic intake, we look at all the symptoms a person has, focusing on mental and emotional symptoms and personal characteristics, as well as the current physical symptoms in order to find the homeopathic remedy that most closely matches the total symptom picture. Homeopathic remedies are made from almost any natural substance. Homeopathy is safe, gentle, and effective. It can be used during pregnancy, nursing, and even for a newborn baby. It works well in all age groups and we have found it to be one of the most powerful tools for treating illness.

The research of Royal Lee, instrumental in the development of the whole food supplement line I recommend (Standard Process), proved that low dosages of natural, high-quality vitamins and homeopathic remedies regulate metabolism and function better in vivo (within the living) than in large dosages. Homeopathy is used to help stimulate the body's natural functions on the quantum level. Health care providers who use homeopathy recognize that signs and symptoms are indicative of underlying imbalances rather than the symptoms themselves. Treating this underlying cause assists the body to return to the intended homeostatic balance. Symptoms are recognized as messengers whereas an allopathic approach, e.g. as in our modern medical model, merely attempts to suppress symptoms through the use of synthetic chemicals and invasive types of intervention. Homeopathy is safer than herbs, due to the simple fact that overdosing or allergic reactions are obsolete. This makes homeopathy the ideal treatment, especially for ultra-sensitive people. Homeopathy offers a complete pharmacology for today's progressive doctor. Homeopathy uses a non-invasive therapy that reinforces the body's natural pharmacy and bodily functions. It works on the biochemical level where all disorder begins, and it works immediately. Energetic stabilization of ingredients includes the use of sarcodes (healthy tissue), allersodes (to reduce allergic reaction), nosodes (which increase detoxification), and isodes (which produce healing effects). For an example, allergies are addressed by taking a homeopathically prepared remedy to gradually desensitize the system to the allergen, eventually eliminating the allergy rather than suppressing the symptoms.

(Quantum is the level of which the most subtle changes are made, yet most profound. by definintion, quantum means the most minute particle or portion.)

In general, homeopathic remedies can be taken at the same time with other homeopathies but should not be taken with herbal remedies. Of course, keep in good communication with your practitioner when you are uncertain.

Hahnemann believed that the parents' basic lifestyle, their emotional condition and habitual diet, and even the atmospheric conditions at the time of conception would affect the quantity and severity of miasms passed on to the child. Miasms are serious disturbances of what homeopaths call the patient's vital force that are inherited from parents at the time of conception. The term *miasm* comes from a Greek word meaning stain or pollution. As in acute prescribing, constitutional prescribing is holistic in that it is intended to treat the patient on the emotional and spiritual levels of his or her being as well as the physical. These are two ways of many that I recommend for family healing. Constitutional also called *classical prescribing*, is a holistic system of remedy-finding. Constitutional prescribing is also aimed at eventual resolution of the health issue, not just suppression or relief of immediate symptoms. The assessment of a constitutional remedy is best done by a professional and other means of the use of homeopathic remedies can be utilized by the purchase of a homeopathic home kit. Such a kit contains the most commonly used/needed homeopathic remedies with a booklet of instruction.

Take control of your own health by recognizing and treating acute ailments quickly using homeopathy. Although It is always advised to seek a trained professional for best results, regardless homeopathy serves as a very cost-effective form or healthcare that is 100% safe. It is forgiving, meaning that you can take it without negative effects if mis-used. Refer to the Homeopathy Tipsheet at the end of this book.

I use homeopathic Cell Salts and a custom blend I make for myself often. I believe Cell Salts have been a lifesaver for my family members on a couple of occasions. Cell Salts are the minerals our body uses the most and taking the homeopathic form instantaneously balances our system.

I'll share a personal story with you regarding the emergency application of homeopathic Cell Salts. It was just before my daughter's first birthday; she had taken a hard fall. She stopped breathing and her nervous system seized; she became stiff and her eyes rolled back in her head. Her older brother ran to get the remedies as I instructed him to. He then called 911 and performed amazingly on the phone at his tender age of six. I dropped the homeopathic formula into my baby's mouth, gave her little body a couple breaths and she came back to us. I always carried these emergency remedies wherever we went. A bottle was kept in the kitchen, diaper bag and I still carry them in my purse today.

A product called Epimune is a very effective immune support. It is a vegetarian supplement and is designed as a comprehensive supplement, meaning that it can be taken as a main nutritional. I recommend switching between Catalyn and Epimune seasonally. Epimune is a fermented product using Saccharomyces cerevisiae, beta-glucans, Mannan-oligosaccharides, nucleotides, amino acids and other nutrients. It contains Maitake Gold mushroom (there is no other mushroom studied as much— over 500 studies), Turkey Tail mushroom (caution: this product is NOT for those with allergies to fungus), Calcium lactate and Acerola cherry for the source of Vitamin C and Zinc. This is a very potent product, only two capsules a day is needed.

When it comes to the immune system, I must take this opportunity to speak of calcium. It is not spoken of much in relation to immunity, but it is essential. If you had enough calcium, you would ward off everything; your immunity would be strong and it is said that you would never fall ill if your system had sufficient amounts of this important mineral; however, it is important not to supplement with just any form of calcium! As stated in the description of Calcium Lactate in the NutriTec software I use to provide clients with the descriptions of recommended supplements: "Although more calcium supplements are sold than any other mineral, most are poorly absorbed from the gastrointestinal tract into the blood." Calcium lactate is indicated for use where there is rapid heart rate, muscle cramps, nosebleeds, excessive menses and for the uterus in general, bleeding gums, excessive salivation and mucus secretion, fevers, tremors and hyperirritability. The mineral calcium is lost rapidly during times of stress. Emotional signals that tell you of a potential deficiency include nervousness or anxiety and irritability, especially in children. Babies should never have teething pain; it is a lack of calcium when they do. I recommend calcium lactate, and this is not a dairy product, as it contains no whey or lactose, and is safe for people allergic to milk products. Standard Process' Calcium lactate product is also 1/3 magnesium. Both are critical in muscle contraction, nerve impulse, and blood coagulation.

Botanicals are only advised on an individual basis, that is by a trained professional. Yes, we all should be supplementing with herbal teas and traditional wisdom remedies just as we strive for a well-rounded diet. With that said though, I cannot advise self-application of herbs. They are powerful medicine and should be regarded as such.

Homeopathy, herbal or nutritional supplementation, acupuncture, chiropractic, and other natural therapies, as well as Biofeedback therapies, can produce an initial increase in symptoms or what is known as a healing crisis. These symptoms can feel like the onset of a cold or the flu and may last around three days. Headaches, body aches, slight fever, and perspiration may be some of the symptoms or simply feeling tired and sluggish. It is important to listen to your body and these signs. Rest when you're tired, and drink plenty of purified water. It is advisable to decrease or temporarily eliminate the intake of any foods your system has a hard time digesting. Naturopathic principles welcome these symptoms (to an extent) as part of the healing process. Make sure to communicate any changes in your symptoms to your healthcare professional and if the symptoms last longer than a week. The incomplete recovery from an acute illness such as cold or flu-like symptoms may create long-term complications. It is advised to take systemic or often termed proteolytic/fibrinolytic enzymes during and after an infection, or while there is any inflammation. This form of therapeutic enzymes, as opposed to digestive enzymes, differ in the quantity and type of enzymes. I recommend them in cases brought on by detoxification and natural therapies to assist the body in eliminating toxic residue and enhancing immunity. Enzyme therapy (ET) is effective in any healing process and used by many professional German soccer teams and European countries for sports injuries and various conditions. I utilize ET in the treatment of edema, respiratory problems, urinary tract infections, sinusitis, rheumatic diseases, following radiation therapy, and after surgeries to prevent scar tissue. I recommend adding a bottle to the First Aid cabinet! However, do not use without the advice of your HP, nor in the case of stomach ulcers.

Many suffer from colds and flu much too often. The occurrence of acute illnesses often means the body is trying but failing in eliminating toxic cellular waste that can lead to chronic inflammatory diseases and an overtaxed lymphatic system. Unfortunately, the lack of understanding of what colds and flu really are and how they work on a cellular level poses health threats to those who use allopathic medications. These are laden with toxic chemicals, devastating the gut ecology and diminishing the immune system, only adding to the amount of toxins the body must eliminate. As you probably know, pharmaceuticals are only designed to suppress symptoms, often resulting in chronic conditions. Additives such as colors and flavors are a cocktail of toxic substances best avoided.

The best way to keep the immune system in tiptop shape is to eat well (for your metabolic type) and supplement only with the appropriate nutrition, probiotics and enzymes for digestion and assimilation of nutrients. Cleansing the body often through an HP assisted purification program is an important factor in maintaining health. Humans are hosts for parasites and worms, but the body is usually able to deal with them if the internal environment (I refer to this as the Bio Terrain) is in good condition. When the body is under the effects of a weakened Bio Terrain, parasites are disruptive, dangerous and in rare cases deadly.

Biofeedback reactivity testing indicates the body's response to such pathogens. Through the calibration (connecting the medical device to your electromagnetic field), the biofeedback device shows if the body is burdened with pathogens (resistance). It also shows the state of health in the condition phase (alarm, adaptation, exhaustion), the nervous system based on amperage and the adrenals/willpower based upon voltage. This testing can be performed by sending me a sample of your hair.

The diagram below is based upon an educational series I teach. Essentially, it is a pictograph of the internal environment of health and disease. Much like the *Decline of Health* specified above this pictograph demonstrate the same process as it related to nutritional status.

As you see in the diagram below, the state of the internal environment is dependent upon the 5 pillars. Longevity or the degree of degeneration is determined by the rate of oxidation and state of pH. Food intake and assimilation as well as the body's efficiency in detoxification and elimination of both metabolic waists and exogenous toxins affects regeneration. Regeneration is the body's ability to make new cells. The integrity of new cells requires adequate nutrition.

The Pillars Of Health And Disease

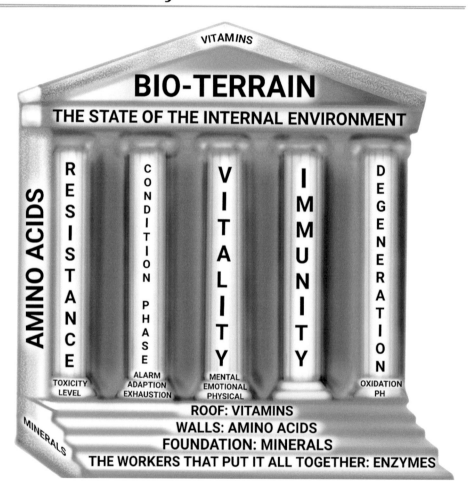

Let healing responses run their course while you rest, drink plenty of fluids, and eat a wide variety of foods per your Ayurvedic Dosha type.

In the case of a healing response, do not stop your program or become discouraged. Protocols may simply need re-adjusted (decreased dosages), temporarily to slow down the response of the release of toxins. Keep in good communication with your healthcare provider who made the recommendations to you. You certainly can increase the speed from any recovery by following the guidance below based in traditional eastern medicine called Ayurveda or Ayurvedic Medicine.

Summary Checklist of Home Remedy Preparedness Kit:

- Homeopathic Cell Salts to use as needed in times of distress, dysregulation, injury or shock
- Homeopathic Remedy Kit
- Congaplex or Epimune for times of compromised immunity
- Calcium Lactate for fevers, muscles aches, irritability, increased heart rate, excessive bleeding
- Enzyme Therapy (inquire about the details)

Other considerations accompanying your kit include the obvious first aid kit. I recommend an herbal salve to replace petroleum-based Neosporin. Silver is another great addition, as it is a good option to use on open wounds and burns. It is also effective against MRSA (a super bug), also referred to as staph infection. Essential oils are also a good addition and have many uses. Do not use essential oils when administering homeopathy. Do not even store the two in the same cabinet or near each other.

Laws of Nature

All too often out of ignorance, ailments develop when we fail to follow such simple wisdom as including all the tastes, (described below) into our diet. The mismanagement of colds, the flu and acute illnesses are one of my pet peeves.

I find that most individuals don't know any better when it comes to the 'how-to' in treating a cold. In desperation for relief of congestion, a cough and lack of sleep, over the counter (OTC) drugs are chosen in hopes of feeling better. What may not be known is that in these very OTC's taken are immune suppressant ingredients ultimately resulting in a decrease of vitality and adding to the body's burden. Dr. William Osler says, "The person who takes medicine must recover twice, once from the disease and once from the medicine."

Usually when you have succumbed to an acute illness, its arrival is to tell you to slow down! Nutritional deficiencies are said to be the basis of all illness and can be in the case of the colds and flu if you get sick more than once a year. However, the causes of the cold and flu are individual. For example, "colds" are very preventable for those individuals that are sugar intolerant or sensitive to food molds (mycotoxins). In these people, fruit is important to reduce or avoid. Particularly apples which often contain the beginning of food mold under the skin. In this case it is wise to obtain the necessary information to prevent and treat sugar/carb and mold sensitivities as this is the cause of most "colds."

Some self-care treatments like putting peroxide in the ears upon first signs of an infectious disease or cold (sneezing, sniffles and tiredness) often will stop it in its tacks! A cold begins in the ears, not in the nose as some presume. Although a silver nasal spray is helpful and recommended during flights (as the circulated air can harbor pathogens), it is far more effective to treat the ears within the first 24 hours of the onset of symptoms. German researchers back in the early 1900's found this treatment to have outstanding results in warding off sickness.

A hot bath with the power of three ingredients will assist you in detoxification; add:

4 cups Epsom salts (magnesium), 1 cup sea salt and ½ cup baking soda to your bath. With the addition of sipping hot tea during your bath, you will have created an in-home sauna like effect. This will heat your core temperature to induce sweating. Just be careful not to overheat and become dehydrated. Liquid Chlorophyll and a homeopathic can

help your body regulate this to make your temperature just right for killing pathogens yet not hot enough to cause your cells damage, this goes for any fever – self-induced or from acute illness. A bath with these three listed ingredients is also an excellent way to kill cancer cells.

After your bath, moisturizing with coconut oil provides a good protection for our first line of defense; the skin. Coconut is also antiviral, an added benefit. Nourishing body butter with the added benefit of essential oils is fabulous. However, essential oils are contraindicated with the use of homeopathy; so choose either one.

In the case of a cold, I would recommend an herbal tea containing Echinacea, mullein that helps restore the mucous membranes, ginseng, and white willow bark with olive leaf, ginger, and yarrow. Raw honey and fresh lemon are also good. The herb fenugreek is very effective at expelling mucus. Use this at the first sign of congestion to prevent a sinus headache.

A diet high in vitamin E, A, D, C, B6, zinc, selenium, and magnesium – as perfectly proportioned in Catalyn and Immuplex. These are whole food-based supplements. The importance in that is to maintain the proper ratio to not upset the delicate balance intended. I highly discourage chemical inoculation of isolated "nutrients." In their deranged isotope, these chemicals do more damage than good and should not be considered "nutrients!" An acute illness is no exception, high amounts of vitamin C, ever so popular to grab for immune support, is not as effective as Immuplex.

The avoidance or elimination of sweet fruits and carbohydrates is advisable in the event of an acute illness. Real foods as in eggs made with bell pepper (contains B6 and are high in vitamin C), mushrooms (excellent source of selenium and vitamin D), onions – known immune supporter, and topped with parsley, or cooked in at the latter part and sprinkled with cayenne pepper (high in vitamin A) are recommended foods. Also, real broths are very nutrient rich, unlike counterfeit broths found in cans and tetra packs and laden with MSG.

Probiotics are a hot topic these days, and rightfully so. However, you should NOT continuously supplement with probiotics because this can lead to a limited gut flora. There are certain metabolic imbalances in which probiotic supplementation is contraindicated, particularly acidophilus. The strain acidophilus generates lactic acid. In some people, the lactic acid builds up in the muscles causing pain. I recommend utilizing a complementary phone consult with me about how to find out what your individual probiotic needs are. I offer a free fifteen-minute phone consult and charge $65 for thirty minutes that includes a follow up email of recommendations.

The use of probiotics, when they are needed therapeutically, is more effective. Therapeutic application of probiotics consists of taking them on an empty stomach about one hour before a meal or two hours after. Regular consumption, at least twice a week at minimum, of fermented foods is ideal. There are some conditions in which this is not advisable and abstaining from such foods along with all vinegars is indicated for some during a period. Such conditions can include, but are not limited to, gastrointestinal conditions and food sensitivities. Again, you can utilize the distance/phone consult option if you have concerns about how to know if you should be supplementing with probiotics or probiotic foods, or not.

Ayurveda has wisdom to offer in many regards. One being in food choices. The concept of food being medicinal plays a valid role in recovery as well as upholds an ideal state of health. By the incorporation of all six tastes (sweet, sour, salty, pungent, bitter and astringent) daily, the variety is provided. The variety in qualities detailed below helps to maintain balance. Each taste has specific therapeutic actions!

The **sweet** taste gives strength to the tissue elements, is good for nourishment, and harmonizes the mind. Sweet tasting foods include rice, ghee and fruits. Sweet food is heavy on digestion. Sugary foods are in no way therapeutic and should be avoided.

Food with a **bitter** taste eliminates bacterial elements; purifying the blood and are light on digestion. Examples include Bitter Gourd, Fenugreek seeds and lemon rind.

The **salty** taste stimulates digestion, clears obstruction in the channels of the body, promotes sweating, and increases the power of digestion, but tends to deplete reproductive secretions. An excess of salt is thought to cause aging and degeneration. However, it is needed to feed the adrenals. Cravings for salt indicate stress and adrenal weakness.

Substances which have a predominance of astringent taste such as potatoes, apples, bitternut leaves, most green vegetables and food containing tannin like tea, possess the properties to heal ulcers and wounds. They dry up moisture and fat in the body and act as water absorbents.

The **sour** taste stimulates the digestive fires and digestive enzymes as with sour-tasting food, for example, lime and tamarind, are easy on digestion and good for the heart (it is only relatively recently that modern dietetics have discovered that vitamin C is good for the heart and it is found in all sour foods). Synthetic sour tastes do not count.

Pungent tastes, as in onion, pepper and garlic help digestion, improve metabolism and dilate channels in the body.

A lack of a balance between the six tastes of food can create aggravation and dis-harmony.

Ayurvedic Foods and Drug Categorizations

1. Tastes (called rasa in Sanskrit) which as explained above, act on different humors.
2. The effect of the potency, (veerya) of the action it has on the body. All food items can be classified as either cold or hot on the body.
3. The last categorization is by the specific effect it will have on the body (prabhava). Two food or drug items may be similar in taste and potency but differ on their special action, for example, figs and dates are sweet and heartening but figs have purgative qualities.

Foods and Balance

Just as machines require an energy source to function, the human body can be thought of in the same way. Think of your body as a dynamic intelligent machine requiring a balance of three different sources of energy. To thrive, the body needs a delicate balance of sleep, nutrients (and water) along with sun to nourish and repair the cells that make up our tissues, organs, etc. Furthermore, there are also subtle energies provided via food and lifestyle choices that also greatly affect us. For example, raw foods verses cooked foods offer different implications. To take a step back, we know that eating too much junk food or sugar depletes our system making us feel tired, cranky or worse! We know that lack of sleep causes all kinds of trouble and we know that stress, over time, takes a toll. Now apply these already known facts to the three energy sources mentioned above. Without going into detail, I would like to create an understanding of why Ayurveda can be a great tool no matter what your body or life is presenting as a perceived problem. This system works to simply facilitate balance. There is great value in gaining an understanding of your own imbalances and taking action to make corrections at the first indication. Only YOU can be the expert of your health. As you tune in more, you will intuit body signals that indicate a need for change. To get started, take the Signs and Symptoms Survey according to your current challenges and/or wellness goals. A fifteen-minute phone consult with me may be enough to direct you. Once you reach a level of body awareness and, in some degree, health, you will be able to manage your wellness through the guidelines outlined within this book and understand when it is time to seek professional guidance. There are the obvious survival needs then there are also these three energy sources or centers that store, maintain, produce, and regulate energy. These three centers are affected by the tangible food and lifestyle choices made, also by thoughts and lifestyle actions.

Without going into detail, I would like to create an understanding of why an evaluation in the imbalances of these energy centers can be a great tool no matter what your body or life is experiencing. It works to simply facilitate balance. There is great value in gaining an understanding

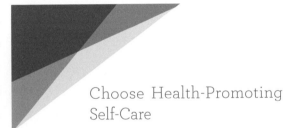

Choose Health-Promoting Self-Care

of your personal imbalances. I believe self-help can only be achieved with this form of awareness. Once understood and having obtained the tools, you can easily assess yourself and gain knowledge of how to create balance.

In my opinion it's all about balance— life, health, and success, that is. Science tells us that everything is made of matter and matter is made up of energy. In all my findings I conclude that current science is only validating what ancient medical systems already employed. The difference is, obviously, in the testing and evaluation procedures. With today's technology, it is very different and has its place and value. However, what has been lost is individualized, natural and intuitive care. There is more to it, but no English word comes to mind when trying to define the main difference. One evaluation I recommend is rooted in Eastern wisdom and called Ayurvedic Medicine.

Ayurveda is considered by many scholars to be the oldest healing science. In Sanskrit, Ayurveda means "the science of life." It originated in India more than 5,000 years ago and is often called the" mother of all healing." It places great emphasis on personalized care according to the individual's constitution. Ayurveda also provides great wisdom on preventive measures and key modalities to utilize in the healing process; some of which include stress management techniques and therapies in the maintenance of health through positive thought processes, diet and lifestyle. Ayurveda is a valuable science to draw from.

Just as everyone has unique characteristics, such as their personality, features, and so on, everyone also has a pattern of energy distinct and individual combinations of attributes. Together, this make-up consists of what is called a *constitution*. This constitution is established by the time of one's birth and remains the same throughout one's life.

Many factors play a part in the make-up and in the change of proportions of the doshas that can result in an imbalanced state. Mental/emotional as well as external/ environmental factors may influence the doshas which can be used to create balance, once recognized as out of balance, for an individual. In other words, everyone has a consistent constitution and certain foods, activities or mental/emotional constructs or exposure can upset your constitution. This is different for each of us, thus the way to restore balance is also.

Energy is required to create movement. In the human body energy is manufactured by the cells (provided enough nutrients) enabling the body to function. Energy is also required to metabolize the nutrients and is called for to lubricate and provide structure. Everyone contains all three components called doshas (respectively named in Ayurveda): Vata is the energy that represents movement, Pitta is the energy of digestion or metabolism and Kapha signifies the energy of lubrication and structure. One of the above three is usually primary, as a dosha. Commonly, a secondary dosha is also prominent. This determines your constitution and thus gives indicators as to susceptibilities as well as self-care treatments to employ when out of balance.

The cause of disease according to Ayurveda is lack of proper cellular function due to an excess or deficiency of one of the three doshas. Disease can also be caused by the presence of toxins. Body, mind and consciousness work together at maintaining balance. In many cases tests (especially blood chemistry tests) reflect an idea that "you're looking good" but you know different. In my practice I utilize today's technology and tests but also apply the ancient wisdom in the treatment plans. Below, you will find both an Ayurvedic Questionnaire and Toxicity Questionnaire (in the back of this book) to self-assess.

Holistically facilitating true change consists of gaining a clear perception of your constitutional state. I encourage you to reflect on the questions below to target the concentration of your personal makeup of doshas.

What category would you describe yourself as being in below (in general) A, B, or C? Make note of the following descriptions in any category that you resonate with the most, then compare each group to see what you notice matches you the most:

Category A: I experience dryness of skin, especially in winter months. My hands and feet are typically cold. I often have difficulty falling asleep or staying asleep. I walk purposely, am outgoing and like to keep active. My energy fluctuates or comes in bursts. I can have a restless mind, but imaginative. My communication is precise, convincing, or direct. By nature, I am anxious or worrisome and my appetite fluctuates. I can be impulsive, or alternately, rigid. At my best I am responsible and self-controlled, positive and creative. My body type (at its best) is thin.

Category B: I sweat easily, often feel hot, appetite is good, and I can eat a lot, but spicy foods can cause an upset stomach. I don't tolerate skipping meals well. I tend to be meticulous and be a perfectionist. I can become irritable or anger quite easily but don't hold grudges. I am usually critical of myself and others. I'm am strong willed; others perceive me as stubborn. I like to splurge on luxuries on occasion. I consider myself to be efficient and disciplined, other say I am intense. I don't tolerate hot weather well. My health aliments consist of tendencies towards skin conditions, ulcers, and other inflammatory conditions. I have a medium build.

Category C: Have a relatively steady energy level, good endurance, and strong stamina. Tend to be slow, methodical, and relaxed, constant appetite, and can skip meals easily. I am a sound sleeper, would love to sleep in, and a slow starter in the mornings. I tend to be reluctant to take on new responsibilities/commitments. I tend to be more frugal and conservative. I am rather susceptible towards congestion/mucus and sinus problems. I have tendency towards being overweight.

Now utilize the tips below pertaining to the above categorization of your predominate type. Often, there are two strong types or, in other words, a dominant one and a secondary. In my practice I compile information into a Report of Findings and detail recommendations in a section called TLC (for Therapeutic Lifestyle Change). You can download food lists for more specific details on foods for your doshic type online or simply have a personalized plan provided though the virtual evaluations you can schedule at virtualhealcareprotal.com

Category A (Vata types):

- Need routine! Consistency brings balance to an overtaxed system. REST is the best cure for Vata types
- Massage daily with sesame oil and essential oils: rose, vanilla, lavender, lemongrass, ginger, ylang ylang, sandalwood, jasmine, cinnamon, bergamot and eucalyptus
- The stone amethyst has a calming effect.
- Color therapy should consist of earth colors that bring groundedness.
- Steam baths, humidifiers, and moisture in general are beneficial.
- Warm, cooked, nourishing and heavy foods are best.
- Spices should not be over-used. Ripe juicy fruits on an empty stomach are fine. Avoid drying fruits such as pomegranate, raw apples, and cranberries. Nightshades and spinach should be avoided in the case of stiff achy joints, or in inflammatory or auto-immune conditions.
- Significant protein is needed.
- A variety of sweet, salty, and sour tastes are important in each meal of consistent times.

Category B (Pita Types):

- Practice virtues of self-control and kindness, generosity, and morality. Avoid heat (saunas/too much sun) and extreme exercise.
- Cooling, calming essential oils are Chamomile, Clary Sage, Cypress, Fennel, Germanium, Lavender, Lemon, and Myrrh.
- Do not over-eat or over-salt. Go easy on the sour and spicy foods.
- Cooling foods and tastes that are sweet, bitter, and astringent are beneficial.
- Massage with sunflower or coconut oils and with essential oils that have a cooling effect and that stimulate sweating: gardenia, rose and improve digestion and normalize energy with chamomile, mint and lavender. Use dry herbal infused oils of yarrow, saffron and St. John's wart.
- The stone moonstone brings awareness and calms the overwhelmed.

Category C (Kapha Types):

- Strong physical exercise is needed. Being a couch potato, consuming sweets, and specifically chocolate, create imbalance.
- Learn to let go of things and not to become overly attached to things or people.
- Massage oils best for Kapha are corn and mustard oil. Deep Tissue massage is very beneficial. Essential oils that are compatible: warming and stimulating: cedar, birch, myrrh, sage, basil, anise and ginger. Strengthening oils of cinnamon, dill, lemongrass. To activate metabolism: cardamom, coriander, chamomile, juniper, sage and eucalyptus.
- No napping, keep active, eat light. Get plenty of sun!
- Avoid fried "heavy" foods, dairy, sweet, tart and sour foods.
- Leafy green should be emphasized. Vegetables that grow above ground (rather than root vegetables) are best. Acceptable in limited amounts astringent and dying fruits are apples, apricots, cranberries, mango, peaches, and pear.

- All spices especially garlic and ginger are very good. Eat a verity of cooked and raw veggies.
- Avoid carbs.

General Characteristics	The Balance	How To Shift
Vata- wind (air and ether)"that which moves things" Represents the nervous system When an individual has this dominant dosha there is a tendency to be thin, light, and enthusiastic, energetic, and changeable	When in balance they are lively and creative; when there is too much movement in the system the person tends to be restless, experience anxiety, insomnia, constipation dry skin, coldness, and has difficulty completing tasks.	Fish and other meat, yogurt, ghee, sesame, ginger, turmeric, coriander, black pepper, cumin all create balance. To decrease- use cinnamon, saffron, fenugreek, and oils To increase- avoid- raw foods, safflower oil, honey, kidney beans and most legumes, mustard greens, pear and banana (especially green).
Pitta-fire and water "that which digests things" Represents inflammation and the removal of waste When Pitta is dominant person tends to be intense, goal oriented, intelligent and have strong appetite for life.	When in balance the person is warm, friendly a good leader and speaker and disciplined. When the fire element is out of balance there is a tendency to be compulsive, irritable, or suffer from inflammatory conditions	Rabbit, chicken, garbanzo and mung beans, coriander, dill greens, radish, pomegranate- create balance. Use a combination of sweet and bitter fruits and vegetables. To decrease- use Ghee, cinnamon, sweet, bitter, and astringent foods To increase avoid grape, mustard greens, celery, anise, dill seeds, ajwain (king's cumin), holy basil, sesame, white mustard and safflower oils.

Kapha-earth and water: "that which holds things" Represents our healing supply of nutrients via blood serum When kapha dominates; there is a tendency to be easy-going, thoughtful, methodical, and nurturing	When balanced a person is supportive, sweet, and stable but when out of balance may experience weight gain, sluggishness, and sinus congestion, constipation and lymph stagnation.	Rabbit, chicken, garbanzos, mung, and kidney beans, ginger, holy basil, coriander, black pepper, cumin, celery, anise, dill seeds, carrot, dill and most greens create balance. Use astringent fruits, bitter and pungent vegetables. To increase- use grape, ripe banana, onion, carrot, mustard greens, chia seeds, flax, pumpkin and sunflower seeds, caster and mustard oils and ghee. To decrease avoid honey, white mustard oil, saffron, fenugreek. I would add red meat here like in the case of a cold, chicken (in moderation) and soups are good, but in general, muscle meat can stress the digestive system, thus creating weakness. I would also add with all of today's convenience foods; concentrated or dried foods. They dehydrate you and create congestion.

Many people familiar with essential oils use them in correspondence with the chakras. While, on the other hand, I find it a more personalized approach to support the constitution of an individual. Attention to chakras can be applied by eating the corresponding color of foods. Additionally, color therapy such as wearing the chakra color, doing art, using lights or visualizations can be effective ways to bring chakras into balance. Essential oils are strong extracts that have therapeutic values such as being warming or cooling. Peppermint, for example is cooling and would upset the Vata constitutional types that need supportive fire element or warming essential oils or more neutral in temperature producing yet having the other qualities such as sweet and soothing (vanilla, sandalwood, rose and bergamot).

From the viewpoint of Ayurvedic medicine, the first step in treatment is to determine your individual type (*prakriti*), akin to a constitutional type. This is determined by the proportion of each dosha that is within each individual.

There are many factors that play a role in your dosha. As with most forms of medicine, this is not an area that should be self-guided especially when it comes to any kind of action taken. However, it can be useful to self-assess how imbalanced you are. With such self-evaluations, you can then gauge how important it is to seek professional guidance and prioritize your health. The form below is something I use in my practice to evaluate imbalances in the psyche. When I use the word "psyche," I intend it as in the spirit sense as opposed to the mind (as it could be interpreted). The essence of who you are is written all over you in various ways. It is imprinted into the way you think and your beliefs, also in the way you carry yourself and the choices you make.

The questionnaire below is colored coded in relation to the chakras. If you are familiar at all with the vedic traditions, you have heard of the spinning wheels known as energy centers or chakras. These questions directly correspond with those centers located along our midline, invisible to the common eye, yet a power source to familiarize yourself with. This is because everything begins in the energy body. Preventative medicines' focus is in the correction of subtle disorder before it accumulates, thus becoming a pathological state presenting sub-clinical or even clinical symptoms of disease. I think we can all agree that is ideal to address imbalances in the subtle level and that it is also easier to correct imbalances than in the more acute stage.

As vehicles for our minds and spirit, our bodies require upkeep in all three areas. They are all interconnected and affect one another. When answering the questions below, average your score based upon all the statements in each section. For example, if you have one out of the three ailments listed in a statement, you will have to decide how prevalent the one out of the three is for you and score it accordingly. Rate the ailment that is relevant to you i.e., the question "I do not have issues with my voice, thyroid, neck or shoulder area." You may not identify with issues involving your throat or be aware of any thyroid problem, but you do have shoulder pain. In this case, evaluate how severe the shoulder pain is and rate that accordingly.

Reflect on the following Questions. Rate how true the following statements are for you from 1-3. One being very little or rarely, and three being most of the time. Feel free to journal!

I feel strongly that I have direction, purpose, and can move forward in life productively and positively.
There is nothing that feels out of control or that is holding me back from accomplishing my goals.
I do not worry about financial security or personal gain more than I should.
My emotions are appropriate to the situation. I feel secure.
I do not suffer from sciatica, hemorrhoids, bowel issues or urinary tract infections.
TOTAL:
I do not feel the need to try and hide or control my feelings.
I live in the present moment and feel connected.
My sexual relationships are mutual and respectful. I am totally comfortable with my partner.
I am told that I understand people and can conceptualize stepping into another's shoes.
I enjoy being creative, musical, or spending time in some form of expression. I have a balanced social life.
I don't find planning ahead, scheduling, or commitments difficult.
I do not have any issues with my reproductive organs or candida.
TOTAL:
I am flexible and spontaneous sometimes.
I do not have many fears or any phobias.

Other's opinions of me rarely affect me more than they should. I do not have difficulty making decisions.
I take on only what I feel comfortable with and do not feel guilty letting others down.
Negative memories do not tend to linger more than they should. I do not struggle with the tendency to hold grudges.
I rarely feel stifled. I do feel I have freedom in my life.
I am not addicted to anything or have issues with blood sugar, cravings, or digestion.
TOTAL:
I can't recall a time that I have had an illegitimate fear of being rejected, hurt, or let down.
I can't say I feel envious or overly wishful of others' things.
I trust without reservation when I know it is safe to do so.
I feel competent in organization and planning.
I feel the ease of freedom from old family values, beliefs/traditions that I have come to realize are unhealthy. Also, I am content with myself.
I feel my sense of self-control is in check, I do not have a weakness in my heart or blood pressure problems. There are no recurring problems with my arms or wrists nor issues with my lungs or breathing.
TOTAL:
I am confident in verbalizing my thoughts and generally feel valued.
I am not overly concerned with financial security.
I don't have difficulty communicating, I am not shy, nor do I over-dominate conversations or have a nervous talk.
I trust my intuition and insights.
I can release any fears and anxieties that arise and do not hang on to negative thoughts.

I do not have issues with my voice, thyroid, neck or shoulder area.
TOTAL:
I can balance my imagination and fantasy realm with reality.
I don't tend to feel lonely or too often depressed.
I am able to give myself credit.
I consider myself to be insightful and have creative solution-finding skills.
I do not suffer from memory or eye problems, sinus or other head related issues often.
TOTAL:
I feel spiritual and am able to call upon it.
I do not rely solely on my own abilities.
I trust in the divine and feel a peace about my spiritual security.
I do not experience headaches, conditions of the nervous system or mental illness.
TOTAL:

Inner Work

The colored form above categorizes the chakras or energy centers. If your total score is above 80 with a minimum of 9 in each category, you are unblocked thus balanced. If not, this is normal however, corrective action should be taken. To start, choose the area (colored section) in which you scored the lowest and put some focus on that area of life that it resembles for you based on the statements. Do you recognize where improvements can be made? Perhaps a good friend, mentor or your partner can assist you in this discovery process. Furthermore, see below for detailed information about the chakras and what they represent in our lives. This section also details therapeutic action that can be taken to create a balance or resolution to issues pertaining to the chakra.

Root Chakra Therapy

"Security is mostly a superstition.
It does not exist in nature, nor do the children of men as a whole experience it.
Avoiding danger is no safer in the long run than outright exposure.
Life is either a daring adventure or nothing."

- Helen Keller

The root chakra lesson is about the right to be, your very existence. Also, it is about lessons relating to the material world we live in; therefore, issues revolving around survival are present when this is indicated as a need for balance. Survival can bring about feelings of insecurity and having to stand up for one's self. Worries of finances and the burdens of society will off-set this energy center. Allow quiet time to restore your reserves of energy and relax. It is important to take time to yourself in meditation/prayer and focus on feeling well grounded and rooted in purpose. Envision feeling a sense of security and safety. It is also important to trust that you are provided for and always will be. Develop and utilize affirmations such as, "Everything works out in my favor I am safe and secure. I love my body and trust in its wisdom. I am immersed in abundance." Evaluate your core needs (see below).

Consider the beliefs you inherited from your environment... do these beliefs still have authority over you? If so, would it prevent you from getting along with your family if you had different beliefs? Is there anything that needs some healing around family? Make a list of all the blessings that you feel come from your family then imagine healing in the areas that need it. Maybe write someone a letter. You can choose to either give it to them or not, but the healing part works the same.

"Let me assert my firm belief that the only thing we have to fear is...fear itself."

-Franklin Roosevelt

Sacral/Navel Chakra Therapy

In laughter, we transcend our predicaments.

-Allen Klein

The lesson here is about the right to feel. Connect to your senses; aromatherapy, burn candles, have a massage, etc. It is important to assert healthy social and intimacy boundaries. Do something special for yourself and refuse to be guilty! Spend time and energy fulfilling YOUR needs. Be creative. You are important and it is important to think of yourself in this way. If it is foreign to you, start by a daily reflection of your creative abilities such as problem solving, in conversation, the way you see things differently from others. Being creative is far more dynamic than being artistic. Become comfortable with your sexuality if you are in a safe and respectful relationship. Find ways to nourish yourself and your desires because you are worthy! Transmute negative thoughts into positive ones. Reframe your thoughts by getting them out on paper, finding your core need in that moment, thinking of ways to give it to yourself then restating the original thought in positive terms. For example, if you find yourself critical of others, consistently crumbing on them, evaluate why. Why are you needing to focus your negativity and project it onto others? Does your core need to be accepted and feel liked, do you need that a little more right now? What else could it be? Form an affirmation around your need such as "I am likable" ... and let it be; so, it is.

Consider your personal code of honor. What ethics need tightened up or maybe you need to become lighter on yourself in an area? What goals do you have for yourself that you have yet to pursue? What stands in the way? Does money have authority over you? Do you make compromises that undermine your values in exchange for financial security?

Do you engage in power plays? Do you emphasize "facts" to support your point of view? Do you use your creative energy in negative paths of expression? Challenge yourself to define your idea of creative and contrast it with other people's ideas. Find the balance in the way you express yourself, in the ways you think and form opinions. This openness will likely bring closeness to your significant other if you are genuine about it (and the energy of it lasts more than a moment and more like a true shift that is palpable for a couple weeks).

Solar Plexus Chakra Therapy

Act in such a way that the totality of your will can always simultaneously serve as the foundation for law-making general.

-Immanuel Kant

Third Chakra work is about finding your personal power within yourself. It is also about balancing the intellect and ego. Let things go more often. Have humor. If you're a naturally talkative person and used to dominating most conversations, hold back and force yourself to listen, without interrupting, to what one of your close friends or family members are saying. This is about putting aside the ego self. Alternately, if you are too quiet, speak up more, assert yourself with confidence (in the right moments, of course). Do things to bring balance to both your creative side and intellect. Find your wit or inhibit it – do whatever is most needed. Mantras you can repeat include, "I am more than capable to ...., I can laugh it off when things are less than perfect."

You have the power to be confidently yourself, self-assured, and successful when you channel the energy of a balanced Solar Plexus Chakra. Those with a thriving third energy center find that they can laugh off their own mistakes, bounce back from failure, and shake off self-doubt. They have an appreciation for their unique skills, enabling them to form achievable goals.

Ask yourself the following questions in two ways, one from an "I think" and the other from "I feel."

How well do I like myself? Am I doing anything active to change what I'd like to improve? Am I able to admit when I am wrong? Am I honest 100% of the time with myself and others? Do I need approval from others? Do I respect myself? Can I stick to my commitments? Am I afraid of responsibility?

Journal these above things. You will be amazed at what comes out.

Heart Chakra Therapy

> *Any part of ourselves that we do not love will revolt. Any part of ourselves that we do not love, we may dislike in another. "We see things not as they are, but as we are."*
> *- H.M. Tomlinson –*

Being about relationships, the Heart Chakra cannot become open without a great deal of compassion and forgiveness. Commitment to mending resolution is needed in order to move forward in healthy ways. This center is also about your emotional power. What emotional memories need healing? Hold this image in your heart. Encircle the situation with a bubble of green light. This is the healing energy. Set an intention such as one that will not allow yourself to be controlled by others anymore.

Try writing a letter to the person with whom resolve is needed, whether it is by you that needs forgiven or visa versa. Expressing how their actions made you feel and lending forgiveness and at the same time letting them know what your needs are is sometimes all it takes. At times, not even giving the letter to them helps you gain a sense of resolve you needed. Fostering of self-love, colorful relationships, connection with others are what makes for happier individuals. Past wounds can begin to heal as they are permeated with positive, Heart Chakra energy. Take some time to invest in your heart's natural capacity to love and have compassion. This will improve your ability to give and receive in loving relationships. Affirmation examples include, "I am love and light, I lend compassion to those around me and love them without reserve."

People with a healthy fourth chakra center accept themselves, can move beyond feelings of vulnerability or regret and recognize that they deserve love.

Throat Chakra Therapy

> *Altruism is one of the glories of our human culture, and it must be learned just as we learn a language.*
>
> *-Sir John Eccles*

The Throat chakra is also about relationships, specifically about communication. Healing the Throat Chakra is about learning to trust and express your beliefs with willpower. Become more comfortable sharing by verbalizing your thoughts to close ones. Spend some time to go within and develop desires then express them verbally. Statements beginning with, "I think," "I believe," and "I want" can help get you started. Similarly, singing out loud (in the shower is a great way to hear the power of your voice). For those who find difficulty listening, it's necessary to first become comfortable with silence.

Others will open to you when you can remain quiet for a period. The practice of becoming comfortable with silence is simple and can be achieved through mindfulness. Being true to yourself takes many shapes. Consider your time spent with friends and what you do in your free time. Make adjustments if the quality of people or activities you engage with do not match your ideals. Mantras for the throat chakra can be, "I can trust...., I am a reliable, good friend, "I can organize and plan for..."

Contemplate if you feel you truly deserve healthy relationships... why or why not? What fears do you have that prevent you from becoming emotionally whole and healthy? Do you know what needs to change within yourself but inevitably put off taking action? Identify what your reasons are. Once you do this you will begin to break down the barriers that you've been hiding behind. The imagination of how it would be to overcome the above brings you one step closer to getting there.

I measure the strength of a spirit by how much truth it can take.

Friedrick Nietzsche

Third Eye Chakra Therapy

The wise try to adjust themselves to the truth, while fools try to adjust the truth to themselves.
Thibau

Seeing clearly, living with clairty, and knowing truth comes form this very important energy center – the 3rd Eye. It is about our relationship to self and spirit; put simply-intuition. It is also about mental power. The spiritual lesson here is about your ability to "see", and additionally - trusting in your own insights. Tension accumulates up in the forehead, at the location of Third Eye Chakra, when we ignore the intuitive voice. To access your own perceptive powers, try bringing your awareness to the Third Eye Chakra center. Developing psychic abilities and self-realization happens when we use this intuitive power. Delving deeper into your inner self may come more difficult than you might imagine. A great visualization technique that increases your sense of intuition is to close your eyes and see yourself doing something you'd like to accomplish.

Keeping a dream journal where you catalog your night dreams allows you to tap into your subconscious mind. Animals or symbols in your dreams come to guide you to use their power attributes.

Change attitudes that disempower you. You can make a shift about what you know isn't true about yourself with words of affirmations. A good technique to identify what your core needs is to visualize yourself in a moment of great need, perhaps as a helpless child or feeling vulnerable in a time as an adult... what did you need to hear? How could someone reassure you? Now, become that person, either a grandmother figure or a wiser older version of yourself, simply telling yourself that you'll make it, it's going to be okay, or whatever it is you needed to hear back then. This helps you repair the core need you had and move on from that point now having the self-assurance that maybe you'd been lacking. Carrying around this sense of lack unconsciously leads us to leverage self-talk and limiting thoughts about ourselves. No more making excuses! Live consciously and do the above exercises to resolve the past.

Crown Chakra Therapy

Becoming human means discovering our fullness and learning to live from it. This involves bringing forth more of who we really are and becoming more available to whatever life presents.

-John Welwood

Whether or not we choose to acknowledge it, we are all given the gift of spirituality. This spirituality defines our sense of connection to a creator who may take one of many forms depending on our personal or religious beliefs. Whatever your beliefs, your Crown Chakra center connects you to your higher self by integrating the energy from all six chakras. When we fail to cultivate divine consciousness, this seventh chakra center can become closed. When this happens, feelings of aloneness and isolation prevail, and life can seem like a series of meaningless, unconnected events. It can be extremely hard to make sense of suffering without a link to the divine.

The events that shape our lives also form the foundation for faith, where suffering can challenge one's beliefs. If you're skeptical of any kind of divine presence in your life, and reluctant to say you believe in a God, ask yourself why. Do you have lingering anger or a sense of dejection that is driving your sentiments? Addressing those feelings can help you open your Crown Chakra so you can begin to feel a connection to a holy presence. Any time that you call to mind your higher self, whether it is through prayer or silent meditation, you are nurturing the energy of your Crown Chakra. Spiritual sustenance can take the form of a religious ceremony, a yoga practice, reading a holy text, an act of charity, or an imagined conversation with your creator. The key idea is to address your own spirituality, instead of ignoring its existence. You can get started today by repeating these positive affirmations out loud:

- I am connected to my higher self.
- Divine power flows through me.
- I speak my highest truth.
- I am a spiritual being.
- There is a presence guiding me through life.
- I am never alone.

Once you've recognized a divine connection through the Crown Chakra, you can stop worrying about the problems you may face in life. Those that have an open seventh chakra do not feel as though they must bear their worldly burdens alone – they truly believe that someone is watching over them throughout life. The faith that is quarried from the Crown Chakra center is unshakable and prevails even throughout times of extreme suffering or pain. Alongside this faith, there is an overwhelming sense of gratitude for each blessing that is experienced. Day-to-day life is made precious by virtue of an omnipotent presence underlying each action. When you're ready to accept this presence into your life, devote some time each day to drawing your attention to the Crown Chakra energy center.

Repeat this affirmation for spiritual wellbeing: *All is well within my soul.*

Below is a list of an essential starting point or reminder to be cognizant of:

The Hierarchy in Achieving True and Lasting Health

1. Integrate spirituality into your life *daily.*
2. Mind-set matters! Commit to positive mental views — this includes filtering your input of media!
3. Establish healthy relationships that hold you to your values.
4. Be physically active regularly.
5. Choose health-promoting whole foods. Simply eat to support your body.

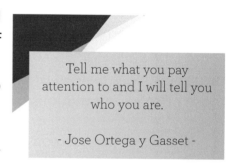

Tell me what you pay attention to and I will tell you who you are.

- Jose Ortega y Gasset -

The list above is your healthy lifestyle focus in successive order. If thoughts follow what perpetuates in the physical realm, then we must first address the mental and emotional interplay. Stress reduction, focused awareness and visualization techniques can be a tool in healing.

In my practice, I offer what I call In Sync sessions or Immersion classes. They are designed to support the energetic body with biofeedback therapies that work to "tune" and ground you into a state of health energetically. This works to stimulate the physical body providing it is the resonance it can align with. For those who cannot attend sessions locally, I offer a body tuning program called Harmonic Energetic Balancing (HEB). The HEB is a program which sends you harmonizing frequencies of colors, among other balancing frequencies, that balance the chakras and other therapeutic energy signatures of the earth creating stabilization of your energy field. This ancient wisdom merged with cutting edge technology provides perhaps the most transformative tool on the planet.

The effects on this level can be felt into the physical body because all imbalances begin in the energetic and emotional body. As it is cleared and healed there, physical symptoms can begin to dissipate. These frequencies bathe the holographic image of the HEB members throughout the day and night, neutralizing, detoxifying and harmonizing. The ancient practice of the Prayer Wheel in which a monk spins with prayers written on it, is said to increase the power of the prayer. This has shown to be effective in many studies, namely The Intention Experiment. The HEB computer-based program is said to be "as if having 100 Tibetan Monks praying for you 24/7!"

Energy medicine works with the electromagnetic field. Because the space between cells is the energy field that makes up our bio-energetic state of health, this energy field can be positively affected without distance being a barrier. The work that I do around the energy body, whether that be through biofeedback therapy or otherwise, I believe contributes greatly to what it referred to as having vagal tone. The term "vagal tone" refers to the regulation of part of the nervous system called the vagus nerve.

The word vagus literally translates to "wandering" in Latin. The vagus nerve is the longest and most complex of all the cranial nerves, beginning in the brain stem behind the ears and then wandering down the sides of the neck, throughout the chest area and ending in the lower abdominal region. While some nerves have either sensory or motor functions, the vagus nerve has both. Motor and sensory fibers branch out from the heart, gut and lungs to other areas including the gallbladder, spleen, liver, kidneys and beyond. This complex nerve affects the entire body and there is a growing body of evidence supporting the use of various therapies and techniques aimed at stimulating the vagus nerve to target specific conditions and stress disorders as well as for overall health. Improving vagal tone benifits the physiology as well as psychological wellbeing. Because the gut is considered the second brain—being that it produces neurotransmitters previously thought only to be made in brain tissue—the vagus nerve has a large impact on mental health issues including anxiety, depression and more.

Stimulation of the vagus nerve directly through biofeedback therapy results in having more vagal tone. The more "vagal tone" we have, the better we can handle stress, experience fewer digestive problems and other physical issues. We are more mentally and emotionally balanced. The vagus nerve is the main player of the parasympathetic nervous system (rest and digest) versus the sympathetic branch (flight or fight) of the nervous system. Absorption of nutrients, by the release of intrinsic factors the vagus nerve is responsible for, is vital for digestive efficiency from the stomach to the colon.

"Indirect stimulation" of the vagus nerve through breath work is one of the most effective ways to bring calming to your system on your own. Because we do not have conscious control over the parasympathetic branch of the nervous system, deep breathing is considered indirect stimulation. The exhalation phase of breath work causes the heart rate to decrease. Alternately, inhalation causes the heart to beat faster in order for oxygenated blood to circulate throughout the body.

We can visualize the heart working this way to stay focused during breath work. Some studies suggest that the vagus nerve is what allows us to get into a mental state of "flow" which can be activated through singing (nihgov). Meditation is also an ideal way to increase vagal tone. Studies consistently show meditators have an overall increase in positive emotions, like joy, interest, amusement, serenity and hope. Prayer and laughter also induce good vagal toning effects. Studies have found that higher vagal tone is associated with greater closeness to others and more altruistic behavior (psychologicalscience.org, n.d.).

The vagus nerve and parasympathetic nervous system are responsible for bringing the body back to homeostasis, or to a state of balance, after periods of stress and anxiety. *Psychology Today* points this out in an article entitled, *A Vagus Nerve Survival Guide to Combat Fight-or-Flight Urges.* "Unfortunately, the Toffleresque 'future shock' of the 21st-century digital age (marked by too much change in too short a time) is causing our evolutionary biology to short-circuit by throwing our individual and collective nervous systems out of balance," writes article author Christopher Bergland.

We can counter this "future shock" by making biofeedback therapy a priority, joining a yoga class or walking club, scheduling time in nature, and getting regular craniosacral therapy and/or bodywork. Additionally, the work below can serve to integrate experiences, good or bad. Integration, or a way to process our experiences, helps us to move through challenging situations in a healthier way.

Selfcare, Daily Flow and Managing Stress

I have the best days when I begin it with a twenty-minute meditation. Breathing exercises to lead your day, implementing breath awareness throughout the day, and with an evening closing adds great benefit to the quality of your life. I begin meditations with a breathing technique called alternate nostril pranayama. There are short YouTube videos I would recommend looking up. I believe this is a great way to balance the left and right side of the brain and sync your brain with your body. This is due to the alternating of nostrils with the breath. Just a few breaths of this is very grounding and peace-inducing; more so than any other technique in my findings.

> You should sit in meditation for twenty minutes every day - unless you're too busy - then you should sit for an hour.
>
> - Old Zen adage -

Wherever you are on the path of discovery and whatever kind of healing needs to begin, know that you are on the right track. The beauty of this journey is finding your true self, so much more than the person you have been indoctrinated by society of believe you are. These simple steps outlined below allow you to cultivate your power and true nature. Stress and anxiety will bounce off you and you will come into your purpose, gifts and talents to use for the highest good – this is resilience!

The growth you will experience is more than you would through worldly personal-growth techniques like visualization and goal setting. While there are benefits to such, typical means of visualization and setting goals usually stops at the daydream stage. It is a necessary first step, and daydreaming is relaxing, inspiring and stress relieving yet very rarely does it yield results.

Following the steps below towards a rhythm in your life aids you on multiple layers. You will experience deep cellular changes in following the daily flow. I won't go into detail in this format, rather invite you to a personal session. You can book a free session online with me. If you haven't recently spent time dreaming up your desires and becoming clear on what it is that you in fact do want in life, skip down to the Dream section.

Although I struggle with a devastating set of events occurring in my live, nevertheless I continue to choose healthy, happy, life-promoting things to listen to, read and surround myself with. In doing so, the inspiration needed to complete this book kept the flame burning. Despite arduous tasks at hand and emotionally draining topics I must face, time after time, I use the below principles to keep in a mental/

Where there is consciousness, connection flows... evaluate whether or not your attention of mind is life supporting or draining.

Are your relationships supportive and hold you to higher standards?

Is your choice of music uplifting in a pure way?
Do other forms or media provide you a sense of value, security and peace?

Do your food choices sustain energy that is from health-promoting quality foods or merely provide calories?

If physical choices support your aim, these three above areas of "connectors" are like a conduit that can only transmute the same frequency of its connected source.

Up-level your frequency to attune to the highest good.

emotional space of health, balance and even inspiration. I'll give you my current example of the three connectors serving as the prime component in my ability to finish this book. I've used these principles I share with you as leverage to thrive because I choose to, rather than to self-destruct (what other options are there?). My philosophy is that when we heal ourselves, we work to heal others as well. This is so because of the energetic matrix. Someday I may share the events of a horrific atrocity occurring with my family, but for now – know that if I endure tragic reoccurring trauma and abuse of the system not helping me protect my children from harm, continue work and care for myself while the darkest of dark are after me, you can also!

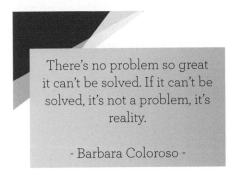

There's no problem so great it can't be solved. If it can't be solved, it's not a problem, it's reality.

- Barbara Coloroso -

Daily Buildup to Rhythm

Level One: Get enough sleep and quality food. In order to achieve these two things, you must have your stress level in check. Get the help you need if you can't manage it yourself. Any form of body balancing you can do is beneficial; acupuncture, massage with chakra balancing, singing bowls. Fortunately, I have a biofeedback device and run myself on the Harmonic Energetic Balancing program. I don't think I would have made it this far without these healing modalities. I also play signing bowls and join groups that incorporate this Tibetan sound healing with the bowls into the group therapy sessions. My deep caring friendships and connection to family as well as my counselor play a large role in my state of health. Having all these avenues of accountability checking in with me, making sure

I do all the hard things I must do, is of great help. I have also learned to ask for help; this is something you must change your mind about if you thought of receiving help from others as a weakness, as I did. It is the greatest blessing, usually for both parties. It wasn't until later in life, I learned about Christianity in a sense of charity work and leaning into one another. Because I wasn't raised in a church-going family and had very little exposure/knowledge of it, I wasn't exposed to the concept of people helping people... it sounds funny when I put it that way, but really; humans are made to be in connection with each other. To serve more than ourselves is something that is very healthy.

Once you master the ability to sleep well (and enough) and consume good food because your stress is managed well, you are ready to graduate to the next level. I must clarify the statement "because your stress is managed well." If you think about it, people that do not sleep well usually have unresolved stress. This could be a literal stress, as in muscle tension. Furthermore, think of the excuses people come up with as to the reason they don't eat well... too much stress, not enough time, etc.

I find that the following order (in levels) is how to build up to the ideal daily rhythm of a heathy lifestyle. However, you can choose whatever order feels right to you based on what you are drawn to doing first, then adding in the next thing and so on. For example, you may find that level four (the last level of priority to me) may be what you would like to begin with. Level four is waking up with the sun, or no later than 6am. This lends to productivity, can allow for meditation, writing, planning, etc. It is all relative to the demands your life has on you and what you can realistically do. You'll know best what to start with.

When it comes to moving out of a high level of stress, even though I can't make it go away, I can do self-love practices to ease the effect of stress. Personally, I do this by enjoying nature, walking or riding my bike to do my errands (as much as possible) to get the flow of endorphins and, I meditate. My spiritual work along with self-care practices are key to keeping me going in a positive direction.

Sculpt and breathe life into yourself with daily self-massage. Show care for your body and automatic self-respect just happens. Self-esteem also emerges from within and emanates forth, in time with this practice. Simply make it part of your shower/bathing time. Touch is vital for health and self-touch is a relationship being built that can only result in positivity. This is called abhyanga in Ayurveda. Part of this practice is to induce intuition through body awareness. This is imperative to your growth and transformation. You must learn to tune in to your body. It speaks to you and you should want to listen, for that is preventative medicine! Begin self-massage with long strokes of the limbs and circular motions around the joints. See where your body needs extra attention and give it to yourself. This doesn't have to take longer than 5 minutes but can take up to 20.

Level Two: Mental digestion and reflection is part of the process and, if allowed, will sync your human experience with your soul's lessons/journey.

- Allow your mind to digest the day by spending quiet time, preferably in nature. Limit music, TV and other digital gaming and media exposure.
- Eat a lighter last meal of the day and before 6pm. Digestive fire is strongest early to mid-day. Make this meal (mid-day) your most nutrient dense and most filling.

If you have been at this for some time (the work to gain and/or maintain health), you may have noticed a change in your natural desires such as to drink more pure water, especially first thing in the morning. An effect of change in areas such as defecation may have taken place. If not, put the intention that you will eliminate your bowels before your first meal of the day. This may require tea and some alone time to be carved out. It is great to drink two cups of hot water with fresh lemon after tongue brushing in the morning. These are good habits to ensure a quality of health you will soon appreciate once you notice the difference it brings.

Level Three: There are moments of opportunity for wellness enhancement in Ayurveda where you can activate the natural healing mechanisms.

Tips for Success

Three causes of disease classified by Ayurvedic Medicine
1. Making negligent choices – when you know better but fail to honor body wisdom
2. Disrespecting your senses – overuse (eye strain), miss-use (overeat), neglect (ignore fatigue), or abuse (loud music, noise pollution) of the senses.
3. Living out of rhythm

⚫ Rest when you feel drained – instead of going for the sugar, carbs, comfort food, addictive substances and caffeine. Good afternoon pick-me-ups should include a high fat, high protein meal or snack to curb the unhealthy cravings.

⚫ Do not overeat. Chew – more than you'd like. Do not consume more than a couple ounces of fluids (and, preferably only consume water and herbal teas) with meals as this dilutes the digestive juices. The size of your fist in amount of food is enough (if you want to lose weight). You will find this to be true if you are regularly feeding your body, not over working yourself nor trained to consider "full" in the all-too-often American cultural way of being stuffed. Note that is takes up to 30 minutes for your brain to register "I'm full". By this time, too much food may have already been consumed if you have not chewed well and with adequate relaxation.

⚫ Just 5-20 minutes of movements coordinated with deep belly breathing, will energize you for the day. Create your own morning movement practice. It can include burpees, jumping jacks, sun salutations/yoga, a brisk walk, etc.

⚫ Facing the rising sun in the morning burns off the fog or depression, anxiety and nervous system burnout. Learning about sun salutations (yoga) is a great

Summer builds up heat in blood and liver, end of fall accumulates a buildup of dryness in the lymph, colon and nerves, winter builds up cold and stagnation in the lymph, lungs and fat. Spring adds damp qualities to lymph and stomach. This cycle continues on down the spiral if not cleared my seasonal cleansing and appropriate diet. The above outlined basic principles are a good start to honor the body and wisdom of nature's cycles that support life. Consult with a qualified natural health practitioner for a custom healthcare approach.

start to the day and are very simple – easy enough for most everyone. Or, simply breathing exercises, specifically aji breathing can be energizing.

● Being in silence/mediation and/or prayer is to live a life empowered. This quiet time opens you up to become available to profound insights as you process your experiences, thoughts and emotions. You gain access to inner freedom and see your life as if through other lenses, or outside perspective, that lends answers that come from your higher self because in silence, you are listening... HOW: Set a time (calendar or timer on your phone). Keep the same time every day. This trains you to tap into and align with source. This results in deep tissue repair (studies show meditation is more restful than sleep).

● Live out your day with several breaks. During this time, open your chest by both deep breath and shifting your shoulder back, even squeezing your shoulder blades together. The cause of back tension can actually be the muscles in your chest caused by poor posture. This is also true for lower back pain; the core muscles need to be activated and stretched. Yoga is ideal to create strength while providing gentle stretches activating many muscles in a natural way. If you have a sedentary job, just a few minutes every two hours to get your blood moving with a brisk walk, jumping jacks or some yoga poses to activate muscles of the abdominal area and open the chest will being much balance to your life.

UPDATE YOUR IDEAS THAT ALIGN WITH YOUR NEW MOTIVATIONS. IDEAS FOR TRANSITIONING FROM SCREEN TIME TO REAL TIME:

TAKE AN EVENING WALK, PLAY A GAME WITH FAMILY, OR READ A BOOK OF QUALITY CONTENT

WATCH THE SUNSET AFTER A CANDLE LIT DINNER ONCE A WEEK (YOUR LATEST DINNER ALLOWED)

CHOOSE A GAME YOU CAN PLAY WITH FAMILY OR JOIN A BOOK CLUB WITH A FRIEND.

LEARN A NEW HEALTHY HOBBY THAT YOU CAN INGAUGE IN DURRING FREE TIME

Bonus level: You should awake before 6am. NO SLEEPING IN! Going against your Biorhythm is a fast track to crashing (body burnout, aging, disease). Staying up passed 10pm or sunset for too long leaves you in deficit of energy reserves for the following day. HOW TO: Early to bed, early to rise – simply follow the sun rise and set (within reason, Northern Idaho, where I live, in the winter gets dark around 4pm!). Surrender to your body's internal clock. Wind down by 8pm to prevent a "second wind" and risk of increased appetite. This leads to, and I believe is, the contributing cause in many cases of diabetes and adrenal fatigue (high cortisol at night and low during the day = fatigue). We need cortisol to react to danger, not to an email or "to-do" after 9pm!

The tip sheet below is a good reminder of what to fit into your day. Prioritize the larger sections and add in what you can, when you can. Coming back to look at the tip sheet can be helpful for making all the listed things eventually feasible. Where you put your attention will eventually lead to the fruition of it.

The three steps out lined above are guides. Choose three of the four (with the bonus level) to incorporate. Make these changes in succession; mastering one before the next.

Daily Holistic Lifestyle Tip- Sheet

Hydrate & Eliminate

Set intention

Breathwork and movement (exercise/stretching)

Self -Massage

Awake before the sun/ no later than 6AM

Meditation/Mindfulness

Early to bed

Work throughout your day with ease and in the flow of natural rhythms

Breathwork for Intention Setting

Psychiatrist Carl Jung described the seeing of repetitive numbers as a form of synchronicity; "a meaningful coincidence of two or more events where something other than the probability of chance is involved" (Schiegl). It is said that synchronicity is born of the unconscious and etheric realms.

BREATHWORK & NUMBERS

Because everything is energy and energy is measurable, thus turned into numbers, it is helpful to put some attention here. You may have heard of numerology… without going into detail I will demonstrate how the method can be applied to your daily life. This is a power to draw upon similar to astrology but more simplistic.

You may find that starting your day with the knowledge of what number the date deduces down to will provide you a feeling of purpose. Here is how to calculate the date into a single number:

Say it is the 4th of December. Simply add all individual numbers of the current date: 12/4 (1+2+4= 7)

If your sum equates to a double digit such as the date 12/25 (1+2+2+5=10) or 12/18 (1+2+1+8=12) then simply deduce the sum down to a single digit by adding the sum together individually like so (using the same dates for examples):
12/25 (1+2+2+5=10) a sum of 10 deduces down to 1 (1+0=1)
or 12/18 (1+2+1+8=12) this sum of 12 deduces down to 3 (1+2=3)

There are Master Numbers with special meaning to take into additional consideration:

The number 11 represents the vision
The number 22 combines vision with action
The number 33 offers guidance to the world

I like to take a deep breath every so often throughout my day and even more so to invoke my intentions using a method of counting. In the circumstance that I aim to find resolve in the task at hand, I find it helpful to inhale for the count of 4, hold at the top of my breath for the count of 2 or 3 (whatever feels most appropriate) and exhale for the count of 6. Alternately, when I feel the need for inspiration as well as a reduction in tension, I inhale for the count of 5, hold at the top of my breath for the count of 3, and exhale for the count of 8, also holding the exhalation for the count of 3.

I encourage you to review the meaning of numbers below but before you do, here is how I became intrigued with the incorporation of numbers in my life:

One wakeful night, I lay awake, noticing the 3am train, I am normally oblivious to, break my pondering inquiry: what would be the number most correlating with the traits of being confident...? The number "one" popped into mind. To be one, at the beginning, or young and having naïveté... it most certainly makes courage and confidence more accessible (given no installments of limiting self-views have impacted a person). So, does the number 11 doubly possess the properties of naïve? No, I initially felt. Although, if you expand the number 11 into a path, in forming a mental picture, being on a narrow path, does limit one's perception, not having a Birdseye view... so it does I concluded. And so, it began - the number meditation. With my group of seekers, we chose a number (at random) to feel out, so to speak, for a week at a time. The following is the agreed upon conclusion.

Spiritual meanings of numbers to use in your daily life can keep you inspired. It shouldn't be thought of as some woo-woo, off-base practice, but it certainly can be kept personal. The point of familiarizing yourself with the meanings in numbers is simply to provide you some insight and direction for your day. This makes it more possible to observe the magic unfold for yourself (as in a sense of spirituality, grace, support or the divine). This is a practice of positivity just as it would be in listing things you have gratitude for each day.

The number 1 packs the punch of focus, a straight path with strong will and pure energy, also confidence. The number 1 reflects new beginnings, and transparency, independence, and precision. It indicates a time to exert our talents and shine. Act and start a new venture when you keep seeing the number 1. Always take into consideration the meaning the numbers have for you personally.

So, what do you do now that you know what number the day deduces down to? How can it bring you inspiration?

You can use it as a tool to set the theme for your day. I have been told that utilizing this has made all the difference in their life as far as coming out of a deep depression. I choose to include this topic in the book because of what a profound transformation this tool facilitated.

Using the example above, if the day is a number 1 day, you can set your eyes on a task that required focus and choose to believe that the energy of the day will support you in this. Or perhaps it's about confidence and new beginnings that you see the opportunity to embrace...

Later, I will show you how to bring it all together using your daily planner.

The symbolic or spiritual meaning of number 2 is balance, tact, equality, and duality. The number 2 reflects a quiet power of discernment and indicates the need for planning. The number 2 signals us to choose; always keeping kindness in the forefront of our intentions. Partnerships and any kind of relations with others (both in harmony and rivalry), and communication are at play, calling us to unite with like minds for support.

The number 3 involves enchantment or magic, intuition, fruitfulness, luck and advantage. In the Christian faith, the trinity represents God the father, Jesus the son of God and the Holy Spirit. The number 3 invokes expression, versatility, and creative expression. It is representative of the past, present and future. A 3 in your life may symbolize the need to express yourself or consider your present direction in relation to past events and future goals. The number 3 has the energy of adventure and assurance of cooperation from others whom you may require help. It typically symbolizes reward and success in most undertakings.

The number 4 - you might think of the saying "the four corners of the earth. To make something square is rooted in forthrightness, justice, being even steven. A foundation might be square. Foundational properties consist of having basis for... Four exudes certainty and authoritativeness, also closed mindedness or being boxed in. It can represent stability, justice, the 4 directions, seasons, the 4 elements. The number 4 has a solid feel and resembles order, family and home, potentially signifying the need to get back to your roots... center yourself, or even "plant" yourself. Some say it indicates a need for endurance and perseverance, even persistence, and reminds us to be present in the moment.

The number 5 deals with humanity as in the way we have 5 fingers and toes. Pythagoreans saw it as a symbol of marriage (the sum of 2 being female and 3 being male in quality), travel, adventure, and motion and the highs and lows that can accompany it. Naturally, this can carry a wild energy, instability and unpredictability, also radical changes at times. The number 5 draws our attention to the curiosity of life and beckons us to notice the *perception* of chaos around us. When 5 continues to pop up in your life be prepared for some action or change. Sometimes a getaway, change of direction or an inward journey is in order. Some of the best changes and journeys are taken in the mind and spirit. You may have heard of praying 5 times a day or repeat something 5 times in order to remember it. The number 5 is about making important choices.

The number 6 represents the balance in earthly and heavenly realms. The symbolism behind 6 is of the earth and legend; love, truth and solutions. In mathematics it is considered the "perfect" number. The bible tells of the earth being created in 6 days. We invoke the 6 when we need delicate diplomacy when dealing with sensitive matters with intuition as our guide (having a "sixth sense").

The number 7 engages the esoteric, scholarly aspects of magic, such as shamanism or sorcery. You've heard of "lucky 7," there are 7 colors of the rainbow, 7 days in a week, etc. It has meaning in the phases of human development. It represents the mystery, imagination and manifesting results in our lives through the use of conscious thought and awareness. With a deeper understanding of the aspects of 7, you can utilize its vibration to your advantage.

The number 8 and the symbol of infinity, deals largely with resourcefulness, success, and wealth. Since 8 represents continuation, repetition, and cycles, determination and hard work play a role here. As an equalizer, 8 also represents momentum. There is a healing quality to the number 8 as well.

The number 9: "Cloud 9" refers to "heaven" metaphorically and brings us to the very height of vibrational frequencies in the numerical sequence. This height can be thought of as an omen to take a "bird's eye view." The number 9 represents the higher purpose, attainment, satisfaction, accomplishment, and wisdom. There is also reference to the intellect and influence over situations and things as well as self-examination.

The number 10 represents space, all possible space, completeness and the 10 commandments indicating virtuousness.

The number 11 is a master number. It has a dynamic meaning, first possessing double power of 1, also fulfillment, congruency and higher ideals, intervention or refinement. It can be a sign intended to encourage us to make an urgent change (hence the saying "the eleventh hour"). The Roman equivalent of a police force comprised of 11 men to hunt down criminals. Several teams are made up of 11 participants. It holds both male and female energy, also both the moon and sun energies.

Dreaming and Productivity

Realistically, I would call a successful productive day being the accomplishment of 90% what I tasked myself with. However, I have come to learn that this is narrow-minded. Having this acknowledgement made me contemplate my values, what I view as "successful" and align my soul's purpose with my will, thus altering my to-do's just slightly. I decided to take my intentions to another level. I got to thinking how bogged down my do-to lists made me feel; forever having a ton of things to accomplish. I changed my method. I began taking my lists and transferred the information to sticky notes categorized by themes. I posted them all on a sheet of paper that I kept in my planner. Then, I moved that sheet of paper from my planner where I rarely saw it and onto my wall. I had only looked at it in the planner when I had a moment of time to see what I could check off the to-do list. I found that when it was on the wall, it was as if subconsciously I absorbed the information and integrated it into my world, things just didn't feel as arduous. I felt lighter. I played with a few ways to organize intentions verses goals and integrate them in a planner. I was inspired to develop just the right format for all my ideas that were proving to make me more productive and more intentional about my long-term aspirations, while keeping me in line with who I am. Later, I heard about Rituals for Living Dreambook + Planner. It is a little bit of an investment, but you may find it to be worth it. I decided not to re-invent the wheel. I also find that a regular day planner with pages allowing expansion for writing and intention-setting will do. A separate notebook for journaling and long-range planning is needed as well. This is great to do with your partner or a friend. Schedule in mini-retreats every couple of months to review. I'll give you examples of this and a good time to do this work is during a new moon. You've heard of full moon energy bringing out the wild in us. More crimes happen during full moons, births also increase during full moons. New moon energy provides creative forces and is a good time to make new plans and charge ahead. Try to work with these cycles. It is helpful to consult an online source to follow that will give you astrological updates in your inbox so your consciousness can merge with these energetic forces.

Before getting into the organization of planning, let's give some energy and creative forces to dreaming. Let's begin with the journaling, or at the very least, contemplation of the following questions to develop or expand your ideal self.

In all the areas or domains of life, one thing remains constant; that is your soul's purpose, referred to as your "dharma" (an Ayurvedic term for your soul's purpose). The closer you come to being true to yourself, the more your personal principles or virtues will reflect your dharma. Below is a list and are some examples of what may resonate with you. I would recommend first visualizing who you would like to be at your peak, the ideal version of yourself. Bring in all the senses when doing this visualization. Smell, taste, feel, and hear what it is like to be in your ideal scene... to be your best self...

1. What do you want most in life?
2. To begin, write down the very first thing that comes to mind. Try to identify your ego self vs. your authentic self.
3. Consider your most valued principles. See list below.
4. Think long-range... perhaps about what you would like to have had achieved by the end of your life.
5. What amount of time is spent exploring, creating, or at play?
6. Detail the relationships in your life... How are you nourished and what do you contribute to others?
7. How do you feel in your body?
8. How is the quality of your physical strength, flexibility and physique?
9. What are your ideals on diet, exercise and aging?
10. How do you imagine responding to difficulty?

If this exercise is challenging for you, try it a few times over the course of a couple weeks and refrain from getting discouraged. In any case, working with a professional is always helpful. It also may be that you need to work on the level of self-awareness before you attempt anything involving the dream/fantasy state. You may be in self-sabotage mode and not believing that you are deserving of much more than you have/are at this point. If this sounds like you, skip down to The Journey to Clarity section. Heather Holistics provides Life Purpose Coaching, ideal for this identification process. Biofeedback therapy is also very helpful to clear the energy field and balance energy centers making it easier to do this inner work. A ritual

> THERE IS NOT A MAGIC BULLET FOR SUCCESS BUT THERE IS ONE MAJOR PLAYER THAT MAKES SUCCESS SUSTAINABLE AND THAT IS HAVING CLARITY!

to set the tone, when performing inner work or before journaling and planning for your day or week, is very helpful. Refer to the above breathing exercise.

Domains of Life

Spiritual & Psychological
Well-being

Relationships, Community &
Connection (with nature and
within self)

Physical Fitness

Creativity, Expression,
Enjoyment & Adventure

Livelihood, Career &
Influence

I recommend about an hour set aside without distraction to contemplate, plan, journal and meditate with the goal of only needing about half that time to accomplish the task intended. This reduces anxiety of not having enough time and when you achieve what you intended in 30-40 minutes, you feel pleased to have spare free time! This one-hour slot should be the minimum amount of time set aside for this time of work each week. Initially, in beginning this process of life-evaluation, several hours, perhaps a full weekend can be set aside.

After some determination of your principles based on all domains of life, use the list of principles/virtues below to connect with your desires. Additionally, try to decipher your soul's purpose, with respect and care not to merely make the following determinations of your principles based solely on your desires alone. In other words, you will have most success by aligning to your higher purpose with the emergence of your personal interests, hobbies and overall mindset. Perhaps, you will become motivated to strive in taking care to self-direct in alignment with your newly defined ideals, even dharma.

<u>Principles/Virtues List</u>

Achievement	Expression	Love
Benevolence	Flexibility	Modesty
Beauty	Generosity	Optimism
Community	Honesty	Peace
Compassion	Individuality	Persistence
Courage	Integrity	Respect
Devotion	Justice	Simplicity
Enjoyment	Kindness	Vision
Equality	Lightness	

About Time

As I stated before, my idea of productivity being successful is when I have achieved 90% of what I set out to do. Although I agree with that however, I sometimes must alter my expectations of myself. For instance, due to all my inspirations and projects, I often get sucked into one of them. This is okay because I am still moving forward towards completion of something. It just may happen to mean that 50% of my to-do's didn't get done as I outlined for myself. This should be considered an exception because it is still progress, yet it must be balanced with the other things that also must be done. It's all about balance. Make sure to set realistic standards for yourself in terms of daily tasks. For instance, during times of the completion of a project, limit your list of tasks to do that do not pertain to that project. The balance comes into play when you find yourself neglecting self-care, bills that needs paid on time, etc. A good way to self-assess balance of time, productivity and self-growth all at once is by utilizing the following chart. Before that however, I would like to introduce a concept of balance in four quadrants of life that relate to fulfillment. Fulfillment is a human desire at the most basic level of our drive (unconsciously) and can be an aim we are able to intentionally direct. Having an intentional blueprint of self-fulfillment can help you organize your priorities and manage your time accordingly.

The basic need for financial security is quadrant number one. However, you can't focus all your energy in this one place or relationships suffer, and therefore it is not priority number one. Too much focus on this first quadrant stresses your relationship with yourself as well as others. The second quadrant is service, seemingly opposite to the first quadrant but you may begin to see how the two can complement each other, if you work with your dharma or explore archetypes. This section's topic is dependent on your profession/livelihood and interests. The last two areas of a balanced self-fulfilled life are self-actualization and enjoying the journey we call life - lived out.

When you have balance in all the above quadrants, you feel deeply satisfied. So, let's see how expressing who you are meant to be, moving towards your highest potential version of yourself, within the framework of the other three quadrants of finance, service and the journey can work *for you* with ease. In the following chapter, we will explore the very root of what causes disjointed patterns of behavior and learn to make a conscious choice for the better.

In examination of the above quadrants and perhaps some journaling, it's time to explore how to take what you desire and fashion it into a format that will help you manage your time. This can be an illuminating process of how you are spending your time verses how you could be.

In each box below, fill in the hours (approximately) spent on various tasks, including that which occupies your attention (even if you are not "doing" anything). At first, simply glance at the categories below and fill in whatever floods your mind. Do not try to organize your thoughts just yet. At this stage let inspiration and intuition guide you then you can analyze it more in detail. This can be done in the goal-setting frame of mind, idealistic mindset or to logistically organize your life's tasks with more intentionality. Most people have between 6am-7pm totaling 12 hours that are considered "waking hours" in completion of a day with intent to these purposes.

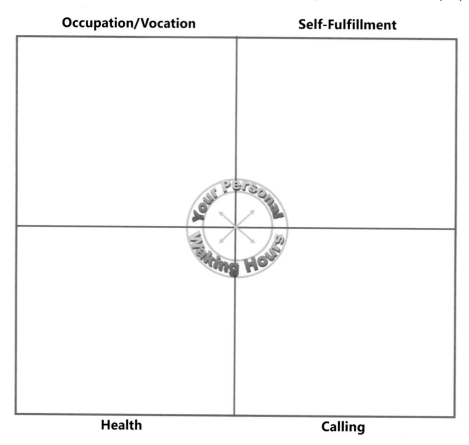

List everything that which occupies your attention (even if you are not "doing" anything). Miscellaneous time spent, such as watching TV goes in the *Self-Fulfillment* box. The arrows in the center indicate that ideally, your occupation or vocation should overlap in theme to your calling. Likewise, self-fulfillment should spill into the health category if you are balanced. Thus, you may benefit from doing one worksheet as your life stands realistically and another to set goals. You can also utilize this chart to divvy up tasks for a week or more. I found it helpful to do a daily goal worksheet and a monthly. The monthly allocates for bill-paying and so-forth.

Now that we have discussed how to dream up your future-self, or ideal version of yourself, and have explored the four quadrants of fulfillment, lets comb through some details.

I spoke earlier about using your calendar as a tool for transformation; okay, I hadn't worded it that way, but believe me – it can be! Let this be your last day of floundering about letting life just happen while you mechanically go through the motions. Lets start with Sunday. It is a good day to plan for the week ahead and map out an outline of how you would like to go about it. Mind you, you may start at any day of the week; the format follows the same process throughout every day of the week. You will see in the diagram below that it gives an example for three days. Within the three-day example, you will find that your day begins with an intention. This can also be a mantra or affirmation if you have the room in your planner to write a little more or have another system. Perhaps you can use a longer affirmation that is written down somewhere else and utilize a separate one, word or short phrase for each day. Affirmations and mantras are usually used long-term rather than changing daily. However, to utilize the idea of positive thought, it is vital for setting the tone for the day! You will see Mid-day Moments; I like to use lunch hour to reflect on my purpose or intent and check in with myself. End your day with gratitude. This format sets you up for a healthy, happy mindset that perpetuates. Over time, you will see big changes in your goals, mindset and what is actually happening in your life. This happens because you are bringing conscious effort to the things you want and are grateful for. The more you focus on these things, the more you will attract.

Sunday	Monday	Tuesday
Use the first section of your planner to write your intention for the day. This can be as simple as "feel the love" or "play"	"Communicate well" *Refrain from using words like "better" such as could be an alternative in the above intention phrase. "Communicate better" indicates that you are poor at it.* **Other examples:** "Be vibrant" "Be innovative" "Exude light"	"Keep strong" "Stay the course" **Other examples:** "Bond/connect" "Be clear"
This section of your planner is for the tasks/appointments e.g. 8 AM drop car off for oil change 9 AM **10 AM** **Etc.**	*Be intentional about the way you phrase your intentions and gratitudes so that you are not putting yourself down. This is easy to do unconsciously.*	
Mid-day Moment of Reflection	A Mid-day Moment can help you refocus on your goals or your overall purpose. Ask yourself if you are spending your time wisely...	You can check in with yourself by asking questions such as: "How do I affect others" or "what do I need to let go of"
1 PM **2 PM** **3 PM** **Etc.**		

The last part of your planner's section should be an account of gratitudes	They can be as simple as your car being ready for pick up from the shop without issue.	"Lunch with friend," or "a surprise un-into friend"

The Journey to Clarity

In short, the Journey to Clarity or JTC's premise is that awareness is EVERYTHING. We inherently operate through societal expectations ingrained in us from childhood. These become limiting beliefs that no longer align with our new-found purpose once we are more consciously living. It is helpful to join a group or enroll in a program for guidance now when you seek a shift in this matter. It is important to identify self-talk and know how to correctly and effectively affirm new beliefs. Re-entrainment exercises assist in the reflection of an idea such as the following:

Choose to trust that whatever the current state you may be in, it is divine – not because it's "God's will," but because YOU, as a soul have chosen it (whether pre-arranged or not, regardless, you are IN IT so EMBRACE it). My #1 secret to health and happiness is, no matter what; embrace it – even the horrific! You will not achieve anything being struck by shock, immobilized by fear and stifled by worry and regrets! Be assured your soul is up for the ride!

Dialectic Behavioral Therapy has exercises around what is called *Radical Acceptance*. Distress Tolerance and Emotional Regulation are more tools to utilize if you are in crisis or lack emotional or psychological well-being. You are a unique irreplaceable gifted spirit. You are in the process of fine tuning your gifts and transferring them into more tangible offerings for our world! I recommend getting a hard copy of the book, *The Four Agreements* (be impeccable with your word, don't take anything personal, don't make assumptions, always do your best) as a quick read. It isn't anything earth shattering, as you may have ascertained from the four listed statements, however it has excellent reminders that work into your field of consciousness and may prove to be more profound than you would expect.

In order to harness total wellbeing, we must be emotionally and mentally healthy. Physical disorder can be a result of suppressed, repressed thoughts and/or experiences not ideally dealt with. The solution then must be to bring these potential aggravators to the surface. Dig up and re-associate negative with positive, and with complete acceptance for the past which brought you to the present, and finally the gratitude for what lies ahead! Forgiveness in outcomes follows naturally with genuine resolution through this process!

To "dig up" the old so the new can be imprinted doesn't have to be hard. Simply become aware of your thoughts and how they make you feel. This is where all the power that you harness comes to the rescue! You can choose how you feel – that is always your power in any given situation. While I predict it would be difficult, if not impossible, to outline self-actualization exercises because it is beyond the scope of this book, I do believe the practice of what I call random thought jotting can be a useful start to re-programming. For instance, say you recognized a thought that created a feeling of lacking and insecurity/self-doubt. Jot it down in a notebook dedicated to this exercise. Write the negative thought/emotion on one side and directly across from it, write a reframing phrase. This is a phrase that takes the reality of that emotion and transforms it into a positive. One of my personal examples is as follows:

I'm not ready... I can't possibly prepare for this.... I'm not made for it. I don't have the skills... I'm panicking... I feel myself freezing.	Instead of shutting down in shock and dismay, I'm going to see this as an opportunity. I get to obtain the skills necessary for this task. I'm going to use the fear and frustration as motivators to find out how to learn what is needed.

You can see from the above example how I chose to use the negative emotion as a launch pad of energy to obtain what was required.

You can also use the below transpersonal writing exercises to journey into yourself, dream, imagine and create. Above, was a list of principles or virtues to contemplate as your personal ethos that resonate with you the most. If you find yourself wanting to explore this more, there is work that can be done around Archetypes that is fascinating as well as therapeutic. I highly recommend utilizing these tools while stress permeates you instead of thinking that you'll have time in the future "when things slow down." This is the very purpose of them – to put into use when you most need the work, so find the time to show yourself this self-respect, care and love.

Write to Heal

This is a three-phase exercise method of writing that is not meant to be done in one setting. However, if both time and endurance allow, go with it. First, set the intention that your higher self and the higher self of those connected to you will benefit. This starts you out on a positive note but don't think that your writing should be all hunky dory – in fact some of the best healings come from the most painfully dark or morose stories.

Now, with pen and paper in hand and an undisturbed area surrounding you, write the first thing that comes to mind on the topic of letting go. If nothing comes to mind quickly, perhaps this is a sign that you would benefit from writing about something you are not willing to let go of. Either way, write in first person. This is about you, for you and only for your eyes, so let it all out. You may wish to do a burning ceremony after this. Doing so can bring closure, certainly resembles letting go and can also stand for renewal.

Secondly, I want you to write to yourself from whomever it is that you need reassurance from, or an apology, or what have you. This is directed to your greatest need. It is best to keep it on the same subject, however it's also best not to force an agenda.

The third phase of this writing exercise is to allow you to step into that other scenario. Whatever it could have been like for the person to write to you, to experience you in the first place... write this portion as if it were firsthand from whomever wrote to you.

After some time with the above exercises and concepts, I hope you choose to use the tools within this book to manage your time more efficiently. Doing so brings awareness around how you are spending your time. It easy to let life fly by. Instead, take more control because you *do* have more control than you might have thought you had! It is my belief that depression is a result of one or both of the following underling causal factors:

- Insufficient nutrition and/or,
- A sense of lack of control, thus stagnant or blocked creativity.

Obviously nutritional deficiencies are a cause of a whole host of problems, and I won't go into detail about how effective nutritional therapy is for the reversal of depression and why it is so because that is not the topic of focus here. When a person feels out of control over their life or destiny, the underlying feel is hopelessness. Once empowered through the feeling of hopelessness, by making simple little changes, big shifts in attitudes begin to happen.

Core Needs

Just in case it didn't jump out at you, the root of behaviors is governed by the thoughts, feelings and beliefs we carry. It may be advantageous for you to form a book club and do this journeying with a group or partner, or you can always join one of the virtual programs or consult with us one on one. I provide you a glimpse of what it looks like to be a participant in the New You Program: visit the link below.

You may be wondering, is your focus and attention all that is needed to obtain and sustain a healthy mindset? The answer is yes and no. Of course, where you invest your attention is the breeding ground for manifesting. However, attention alone is only the starting place. I hope you gathered, from the content of the book thus far, that planning as a component to intending is necessary, along with the excitement of being *into it*. So in essence, the focus of your attention being directed takes some intention and perhaps a little planning in and of itself. You could say that the awareness of your ability to direct focused attention is the commitment to it. That is a great start. Then there is the implementation, of which I have provided ways for self-reflection, self-assessing and mapping out your day to incorporate healthier ways. Before all of this can be effective though, your core beliefs must be addressed. Otherwise, you may be in a self-sabotage pattern and if you have tried other manifestation practices before without much success, this is why. The final component to your success is to really be able to *feel* the way you want to *be*. This is the reason vision or dream boards tend to work. The feelings of the colors combined with images evoke the feelings you are looking to create more of.

My interpretation of my studies, experience and surveys about what the top desires of most everyone comes down to are these three ultimate desires:

LOVE

PURPOSE

HOPE

No matter what a person's values are, or their dharma, we are spiritual beings having a human experience; driven by basic needs. Obviously, we have brains that allow us to reason. Reasoning, in this case deeming one to be capable and competent (in our purpose) is reflective of the head center, whereas the desire to feel valued is in the feeling center (all about love). Lastly, hope is of the body center and is comprised of perceiving one's self to be "in control of their life" or "at peace." According to the Enneagram personality typing, everyone falls into one of these three centers (head, feeling and body) and has all attributes but in varying degrees of dominance. The body center is also termed "belly center." Interestingly enough, in the Vedas (Eastern philosophy or Ayurvedic Medicine), the belly area is the seat of creative energy. This would encompass the above category of hope. So, beyond having our basic needs met as in shelter and food, the core desires for love, purpose and hope are the motivation behind how we operate. I encourage you to work with us, or at the very least, take an online test to determine your personality profile from an Enneagram perspective. It is a way to increase one's awareness thereby applying gained insights as a tool for transformation (what I call doing the transpersonal work). Thinking, feeling and relating are the actions based on basic core desires of humanity (love, purpose and hope).

To be aligned in spirit, mind and body is heaven on earth. Through this achievement, you are freed of the constraints fear has on you. What more can I say? Can you see, after some reflection of this bold statement, that when all centers become balanced, there is no more conflict between one's intuition and how they feel and think? Some spiritual beliefs assert that the only suffering is that which we impose upon ourselves. It is because we doubt ourselves, hold onto fear and lack tools to overcome these internal battles that we become stagnant. In prolonged states of stagnation, our physical bodies become ill.

We all want to feel understood and relate to others. How many of us actually take an active role to seek understanding? By this point in the book, you will have been guided to understand yourself more, and I hope, with compassion. Others with whom you are in relation want the same thing; compassionate understanding. Understanding stems from empathy, having empathy makes you vulnerable... to... that's right — *feeling*.

Many of us may perceive vulnerability as a weakness and strive to avoid it. Yet, think of it this way; how can you be caring, sensitive to other's needs, of service and, at the same time, not be vulnerable? Don't you think it requires openness to be a willing participant in any cooperative effort? Whether this be in the workplace or in deeper connections with others, relational skills are all rooted in vulnerability. To truly grow, one must be open to vulnerability. You must first be honest with yourself, then willing to trust others and be open with them. That is a vital piece and if you do not feel you can create that just yet, find a trusted professional such as a counselor or coach. Another option is to enroll in one of our programs.

It has been shown that those who converse about their circumstances, whether that be a business venture or on the personal side, attract more success and confidence. Likewise, I notice those whom I work with excel at a much more favorable rate towards the vision when they include their family and friends in their wellness endeavor. My children and family members have enjoyed the Enneagram insights as a way to relate.

When we talk to others about our experiences, when we include others in our journey, we get to our end goal faster, and with more ease. We are designed to band together... to co-create, co-exist.... Imagine that! You have a choice to make at this juncture; are you going to let your experiences define you and hold you in a place that makes you feel stuck or are you going to choose to gain wisdom from them? The choice is yours to blossom into some magnificent purposeful being living in alignment with the talents and personal special attributes making it possible to contribute to the whole! Each element of one's personality is a valid aspect. If we do not contrast against each other to see these magnificent attributes come alive, we do not realize our potential. It takes more than self-reflection, journaling and planning to be balanced. We need one another's perspective.

Appendix (Forms Referenced within Book) (Alphabetically):

Allergy Testing – Pulse Assessment

Basal Temperature and Resting Pulse Tests to Measure Thyroid Function

Cleansing

> Annual Detox Protocol-Maintenance

Digestive Health

> Symptoms Chart

Homeopathy Tip Sheet

Leading a Healthy Lifestyle

Nail Indicators of Nutritional Deficiency

The PH Factor

Toxicity Questionnaire

Allergy Testing Pulse Assessment

HOW TO TEST FOR SENSITIVITIES YOURSELF – AT HOME:

It is recommended to take your pulse prior to rising out of bed in the morning. However, this is only accurate if the alarm clock or an adrenal imbalance/adrenalin rush did not occur. If so, lay and rest until completely relaxed before taking your baseline pulse. This could take 10-15 minutes. When you are ready to test for a suspected allergen; take pulse before eating or drinking anything. Forty-five minutes later take pulse again (Note: this is 45 min. after taking 1st pulse. If it takes more than 45 to eat your meal; take your pulse 15 min. after you finish). Do the same for all meals or suspected allergens and use the form below to record you results.

If the pulse raises seven or more beats per minute after ingesting a food, that substance is not agreeable with you. It can also be something in, or on the food such as pesticides, food coloring, flavors, etc., for example, in peanut butter, hydrogenated oils are a common sensitivity.

PULSE ASSESSMENT:

The pulse needs to be taken for a full minute either on the thumb side of the wrist (about 1-2 inches from the palm of the hand) or along either side of the windpipe along the carotid artery. This is normally the easiest to find especially in heavier individuals. The pulse should always be taken with the fingers; never with the thumb. Note any other factors such as exposure to cigarette smoke, if you were startled, stressed, or anything else that may increase pulse. This way the suspected allergen can be re-tested later for more accurate results.

Suspected Allergen   Notes

	Time	Pulse Before	After	
	Time	Pulse Before	After	
	Time	Pulse Before	After	

	Time	Pulse Before	After	
	Time	Pulse Before	After	
	Time	Pulse Before	After	
	Time	Pulse Before	After	
	Time	Pulse Before	After	
	Time	Pulse Before	After	
	Time	Pulse Before	After	

Basal Temperature and Resting Pulse Tests to Measure Thyroid Function

The measurement of body temperature determines sub-clinical hypothyroidism which does not show up in the standard thyroid blood chemistry test. Basal temperature and resting pulse reveal the basic function of the thyroid (its ability to regulate the metabolic furnace of the body to create heat or control temperature).

Your basal temperature, which is the lowest temperature attained by the body during rest, usually during sleep, can be measured immediately after awakening. Note that temperature measured at the time of ovulation in women is somewhat higher by one-half to one whole degree Fahrenheit. Take your digital thermometer with you to bed and set it next to you in an easily reachable spot so temperature can be taken right away under the arm, in the arm pit (axillary temperature) without the need to get up. Do not sleep with excess blankets, an electric blanket, or a room over the temperature of 65 degrees. A consistent reading of 97.6 or below means low thyroid function! Above normal range may indicate infection or an over-active thyroid. The normal range fluctuates slightly during the day. Assuming you sleep at night and are active/alert during the day, a normal range 97.7 to 99.5 should be between the time of 10 am and 6 pm. From 2am to 6am temperature falls to around 97.5. Remember within 24 hours of ovulation temperature increases due to an elevation in progesterone. Temperature could also indicate progesterone and estrogen hormone levels. Progesterone raises temperature as well as blood pressure, and estrogen dominance decreases body temperature and blood pressure. Do not attempt this testing during ovulation! During illness the thyroid is also inhibited. Anti-depressant drugs and anti-anxiety drugs will cause an abnormal rise in your temperature, altering this test.

Another good indicator of low thyroid function is resting pulse. Take your resting pulse (laying down in a calm environment for fifteen minutes and after eating by two hours). Measure your resting pulse for three days and compute the average. The healthy resting pulse should be about 68-77 beats per minute (the national average is around 72), but if your pulse is less than 80, you may have an under-active thyroid. Children have a pulse greater than 100 until around the age of eight when the pulse slows down to around 85. The idea of a slow pulse being healthy is folklore. Some low thyroid people have a high pulse of over 100 beats per minute due to excess adrenaline. These people will have trouble monitoring their temperature because it may not be consistent. The most critical thing to remember is to take pulse at least two hours after eating or drinking anything but water, do not be talking to anyone during the duration of testing, and lay down comfortably with a writing utensil, paper, and timer (no sound, so as not to trigger adrenaline on the second reading). You must lay still for fifteen minutes in order to take a RESTING PULSE!

Measure radial pulse (wrist) or carotid pulse (neck):

Radial Pulse – Place the tips of your index finger and third finger gently on the thumb side of either one of your wrists. You will feel the beats and with the help of a clock, measure the pulse for 15 seconds. Remember the number as you immediately start recounting. Multiply both results by 2 and record.

Carotid Pulse - Place your index fingertips and third fingertips below your jaw, along the windpipe and throat. Hold it gently using the fingertips of first and second finger. Then with the help of a clock, measure the pulse for 15 seconds. Remember the number as you immediately start recounting. Multiply both results by 2 and record.

Temperature a.m., before rising 98° F (optimum). Temperature During Day between 11 a.m. and 3 p.m. 98.6°-99° F and not > 100° F (optimum):

1 _____ 2 _____ 3 _____

Average Temperature _____

Resting Pulse when not eating 85 beats per minute (optimum):

1 _____ 2 _____ 3 _____

Average Pulse _____

Another easy way of detecting an under-active thyroid is taking a resting pulse sitting, then lay down, and take it again after having laid for one minute thirty seconds. If your pulse while sitting is lower than your pulse laying; then you may have low thyroid function.

The fourth test is also an indicator for thyroid function in the way of a nutritional deficiency of iodine. Use Providone iodine to place a dot on the skin of your forearm with a Q-tip (the size of a postage stamp). It is recommended it be on the soft skin of your forearm or abdomen. Fill it in gently, dotting the iodine until the rectangle is filled in. The test is to see how long the iodine stains the skin. If it stains it for 24 hours, there is no need for additional iodine. However, if it soaks in (sometimes within a few minutes for some people, and others a couple of hours) then continue dotting on the iodine. You should start on the wrist and move up the inner arm each day. This provides a new area for the iodine so it doesn't accumulate in the skin, as if it would if applied to the same area for a few consecutive days. Within a week you should be up to the elbow in applying the iodine, then move back down the arm. You can keep applying this until it stains your skin for 24 hours, or you can get some pure iodine (that is clear) and conveniently spray it on. If you use the spray-on technique, use the dark providone iodine once a month to test the need for it. Through the skin is the best way to take iodine. Because iodine is a strong anti-bacterial, it kills the good as well as the bad bacteria in the gut, so it is not advised to take it orally.

Cleansing

Phase 1 – Lymph Cleanse
Take *Lymph Max* or *Lymphatic Detox tincture*. Take 20-30 drops. If you are doing the KI/BL cleanse at the same time, reduce only the Lymph remedy to 15-20 drops but increase to three time per day. Remember not to do the two cleanses at the same time if any kind of infection is present. The Lymph detox should last 2-3 weeks.

Phase 2 – The Kidneys
Kidney Cleanse using my herbal tincture or follow Dr. Clark's recipe on Page 549 of her book, *The Cure for All Diseases*. Drink 4 oz. of fresh squeezed organic lemon juice or buy it in a jar (organic *Santa Cruz*). It is not necessary to drink the lemon juice every day -- although you certainly can -- it only needs to be taken the last 4 days of the cleanse. Take ginger tablets or my remedies *Digestive Aid* or *Purify* with every meal. Take Uva Ursi capsules: one in the morning and two with dinner. Do this for 3-4 weeks. Or,

Scolopendrium tincture for 1-2 weeks. You will need to maintain the herbal remedy for parasites at a dose of 1-3 drops two times per day until you have completed the kidney cleanse.

<u>Phase 3 – The Parasite Cleanse</u>
Complete a 10-20-day parasite cleanse with herbs. If not being evaluated by a health professional, do 20-30 days. It is best to know what kind of parasites you are infested with to better select the herbal blend and duration of cleanse. Have Biofeedback and/or kinesiology testing after the 10 days of herbs to be re-evaluated on the status of the parasites to determine if they have been addressed adequately or if another ten days is needed. You will need to eliminate all meat, dairy, sugar, refined foods etc. (as outlined in the *Therapeutic Diet Plan*). Be sure to take good supplements, as always, get enough protein (see Complete Proteins) and eat plenty of organic fresh veggies. Drink plenty of water! Below is an example of an outlined daily plan.

Cleansing Example Sample Schedule

Complete a 10-20-day parasite cleanse with herbs. Drink plenty of water! Below is an example of an outlined daily plan.

Remember, you cannot effectively cleanse the liver with parasites in it! Phosphoric acid softens the gall stones and should be taken about a week before the liver/gallbladder cleanse.

Parasite Detox Protocol

Sample Supplement Schedule

Product	Description	Upon Arising	*On Empty Stomach	Morning	Lunch	Between Meals**	Dinner
Cell Food* (through Heather Holistics or health food stores)	Drink 8oz. purified water with 8 drops Cell food*	X					
Wormwood Complex (Standard Process) or Para A (Marco Pharma) or Dr. Clark's kit	Herbal remedy to kill pathogens- in room temp water 15 min. before luvos clay, 30 min. before meal		X	X	X		X
Luvos Clay (Marco Pharma)	1 capsule or ½ teaspoon with water to absorb die off and other toxins		X	X	X		X
Fiber Rich Breakfast	15-30 after luvos clay			X			
Body High vitamin/Amino Acid Supplement and Major Mineral Mix	Vitamin smoothie (Body High and/or green food in freshly squeezed juice) Mid-morning snack- at least 1 hr. after clay					X	
*Systemic Enzymes	As directed*		X				
Probiotic's	Good bacteria- before bed						

*Do not take systemic enzymes if you have certain gastrointestinal issues. Consult first to find the correct formula.

Remedies (both regular and extra strength) should be taken in 4 oz warm water on an empty stomach 15 minutes before breakfast, and again 15 minutes before dinner.

Dosage Instruction for Para A herbal tincture:

Day one: Take 6-10 drops
Day Two: Double dosage
Day three: triple form original dosage
Day four: 3 more drops than previous day

Day five: "   "

Day six: Maintain this dosage for the next 4 days

Do liver/GB cleanse right after pathogenic detox. A fudge factor of 4 days is allowed by maintaining dose of 3-6 drops twice daily.

Do liver/GB cleanse right after pathogenic detox. A fudge factor of 4 days is allowed by maintaining dose of 3-6 drops twice daily.

<u>Phase 4 The Flush</u> - Now you are ready to flush the liver and gallbladder! You will need the following:

- 4 Tablespoons Epsom salts
- ½ cup olive oil
- 1 large pink grapefruit (freshly squeezed- about 2/3 cup). Note: grapefruit enhances the effects of medication. If possible, refrain from your regular medications during the cleansing process. Or substitute with fresh lemon juice!
- A 1- quart jar with lid
- A straw - makes it easier to drink
- Sleep aid *(Sooth-Me-Sleepy)*

Start on a day such as Saturday so you will be able to rest the following day. Do not take any medication, or supplements that you can do without; they could inhibit success. Eat a "non-fat" breakfast and lunch such as hot cereal with fruit (no butter or milk). For lunch, consider eating a salad or vegetable soup. Keep in mind *fat* is not bad and should not be avoided under any other circumstances other than this cleanse. Fat contains essential nutrients and serves as an important part of the diet. "Fat intolerance," heart disease, etc., need to be addressed with Enzyme Therapy, not fat avoidance!

<u>The Plan</u>

- Do not eat or drink after 2 pm; ignoring this could make you ill! Prepare 4 servings (for convenience) in a quart jar: Mix 4 Tablespoons of Epsom salts with 3 cups purified (but not distilled) water. Store in the refrigerator. Remember not to eat or drink anything but water!

- 6pm Drink one serving (3/4 cup). If you have not prepared this in advance drink 1 T. of Epsom salts in ¾ cup water. You may add 1/8 teaspoon vitamin C powder for taste.

- 8 pm drink another ¾ cup of Epsom saltwater. Do not be more than 10 minutes early or late; timing is critical for success. Finish what you need to do for the night before you are confined to the toilet!

- 9:45 pm squeeze grapefruit juice until you get at least a ½ cup. Take pulp out with fork. Pour ½ cup olive oil and the grapefruit juice into a quart jar, put lid on and shake until watery -- only fresh grapefruit will do! You may need to visit the bathroom before drinking your mix because you will need to lay down right after drinking it!

- 10 pm drink the mixture standing up and within 5 minutes if possible (the straw helps); 15 minutes is acceptable for the elderly or weak. Also take 30 drops *Soothe Me Sleepy*. Lay down on your right side immediately for at least 20 minutes. You may shift to your back with your head up high on a pillow. You may be able to feel the sensation of stones traveling along the bile ducts like rolling marbles. It is not painful because of the Epsom salts! You may be nauseated, if so, take *Digestive Aid* or *Purifier* remedy, which contains ginger.

- Upon awakening (expect diarrhea) take your third serving of Epsom saltwater unless nauseated or have heartburn, then wait until it's gone. A pinch of baking soda in a couple ounces of water helps the heartburn.

Look at the bowel movement with a flashlight and count the stones! The stones float because of the cholesterol and will be pea green from the bile, or tan cholesterol crystals may float to the top that hadn't yet formed into round balls. You will need approximately 2000 stones before the liver is clean enough to clear up allergies, back pain, or bursitis permanently! You may repeat this cleanse at two-week intervals. As Dr. Clark states, you can dissolve all your kidney stones in 3 weeks but form new ones in three days if you drink tea, cocoa, and phosphate beverages.

- 2 hours later, take your last dose of Epsom saltwater; you may want to go back to bed.
- 2 hours later, you may eat but start out with something light. Juicing fruits and veggies is always good! By dinner time you should feel recovered. Take 30 drops of *Soothe Me Sleepy* in warm water, to help you sleep.

To support your liver in-between detoxifications, you can follow Dr. Clark's recipe for tea or take my herbal remedies. Some find that purchasing the eleven individual herbs (recommended by Dr. Clark) and making a tea to be inconvenient, but if you would rather do it that way, I recommend ordering from Mountain Rose Herbs online (for convenience you can find the link on my website). The crude herbs are organic, and reasonably priced. It is important to select a quality company! Some find tinctures easer, as do I (I'm not fond of tea). Make sure to drink plenty of water, ginger or parsley (fresh) tea throughout each day! Equally good as tincture or tablets, is a remedy consisting of milk thistle seed, turmeric root, and dandelion.

Phase 5 -- Heavy Metal Detox/Bowel Cleanse

Remember **not** to take fiber supplements with nutritional supplements!
A heavy metal detoxification is simple; continue taking supplements (ideal supplementation includes a food-based vitamin/green food), enzyme with every meal, and Probiotic's 30 minutes before breakfast or before bed as long as on an empty stomach.

<u>Sample:</u>

Awake: Take Probiotics and a large glass of water 1-2 hours later, take water, Cellular Defense, Bowel Detox herbal remedy, high fiber cereal, muffin, or bread.

Lunch: Cellular Defense, green food supplement and a healthy meal

Snack: Smoothie with Body High Vitamin/Amino Acid Supplement

Dinner: Cellular Defense, Bowel Detox herbal remedy, green food supplement

*For lead poisoning, chemical exposure, medication, anesthesia and other medications, or any other toxic exposure ask about chelation therapy.

<u>Resistance to treatments may be due to the following:</u>

Heavy metal poisoning: check the hair analysis.
Amoebic gingivitis: spray toothbrush with hydrogen peroxide after every use.
Re-infection: through family members*, partners, pets, water.
*Family members should always administer the same cleansing protocol.

A combination of poor nutrition/nutritional deficiencies and the accumulation of toxins can lead to progressive degeneration, inflammation, and various diseases. With the knowledge of the avenues of elimination (listed below) you are better prepared to addresses any issues in the early stages. It is imperative for a healthy immune system that all the elimination avenues listed next are in good working condition.

Elimination Avenues:

- Lungs/Breath: most gaseous toxins exit the body via the lungs —exercise is important. BE SURE TO BREATH CORRECTLY! Please reference section Breathing, Self-Care, and Managing Stress and Breath Work for Setting an Intention further along in this book.
- Skin/Sweat glands: largest organ of elimination—hydrotherapy, saunas, foot baths, foot detox pads etc. are helpful.
- Bowels: most solid waste exits the body via the bowels—less than one bowel movement a day is not acceptable.
- Liver: performs an array of detoxification functions.
- Kidneys: the filtering of waste through the kidneys is vital (kidneys process about 200 quarts of blood daily!) Do your two KI cleanses a year!
  - Mucous membranes: these dump toxins into the intestines for elimination and control, and parenchymal endothelial balancing of minerals.

Another important factor in a detox protocol is the environment; if the toxic environment is eliminated, the body can excrete much more of the buildup accumulated over the years from the system (avoid pollution, chemicals etc.!). Use all-natural cleaners, cosmetics, etc.

Annual Detox Protocol-Maintenance

This is intended for those who are in good health, have completed the initial four phase series in consecutive order until achieved adequate results, and aim to maintain health. The plan below is an option to guide you through detoxification based on Chinese medicine and natural flow of the seasons.

Winter: Cleanse the Kidneys and Bladder in preparation for liver/gallbladder cleanse in the spring. Herbal tea should consist of juniper berries, corn silk, uva ursi, parsley root, horsetail, hydrangea root, gravel root, and marshmallow, or you can take it in tincture.

Spring: Parasite cleanse followed by the overnight liver/gall bladder detoxification. An effective parasite detox consists of black walnut hull, cloves, and wormwood which is what Dr. Hulda Clark recommends.

Summer: Give rest to the digestive system by fasting. The length of time depends on metabolism and various factors. It is best to consult with your holistic care professional.

Autumn: A good time to focus on and correct breathing, possibly administer herbal remedies for the lungs to expel mucus and may also be a time to fast if constipation or congestion is an issue.

*A heavy metal and/or bowel detox can be administered at any time!

Day to day outline

Day 1 – start lymph detox and possibly KI/BL remedy – Do this for 14 days unless otherwise recommended

Day 15 – If KI/BL cleanse was not done during the Lymph Cleanse; do now for 21 days (unless otherwise directed by professional). If KI/BL & Lymph was done at the same time simply continue taking the Urva Ursi for an additional 7 days.

*General supplementation can be taken though these two cleanses, unless yeast is an issue, then take caprylic acid and Probiotics as directed.

*I find tinctures, in general, to work faster and possibly be more potent when taken directly into the mouth and under the tongue for a couple seconds. Children should take with water; also, warm water evaporates some of the alcohol.

Day 22 - Parasite Tincture in warm water (4oz). This needs to be taken in the warm water for effectiveness (contrary to most tinctures). 20 Days following the Dosage Instructions.

Day 43 - Heavy Metal/Bowel Detox – see different options below and discuss with health care provider. Generally, I have people continue taking the Lovos clay (two capsules in-between meals such as about 2 hrs. after breakfast). Cellular Defense is a good supplement and very easy to take. Put drops into water (if it is not with the Cell Food or any other mineral water) and drink throughout the day. Or take in water after lunch. Additional herbs/supplements need to be evaluated for you based on various factors. You will finish the Lovos clay at about day 38 (that gives you 20 days of 1, 3 times per day for 20 days during Parasite Detox, and 2, one time/day for 30 days for Heavy Metals Detox).

The *Cell Food* product contains oxygen that hydrates the body adequately and assists in killing pathogens. It also contains trace amounts of amino acids, minerals, and enzymes to support cellular integrity. The *Para A* and the *Luvos Clay* are a German protocol for detoxifying pathogens. The herbs in *Para A* have been studied and are known to effectively kill over 100 different kinds of parasites alone. Because of the die off, the *Luvos Clay* is used to absorb both toxins and waste, thus reducing risk of toxemia, thus avoiding severe adverse side effects. Do not use the clay if constipated! This causes toxins to re-circulate and welcomes pathogenic proliferation. The Luvos clay has been used in Germany as a therapy for gastrointestinal elements for over 70 years. In addition to absorbing toxins and pathogens, Luvos Clay is used to treat leaky gut syndrome, diarrhea, colitis, gastric/duodenal ulcers, gas, bloating, and after excess alcohol use. This clay plays an important role in a parasites cleanse. The connective tissue is a passageway for nutrients. It is also a storage place for residue and toxins the body is filtering through. The connective tissue is like glue for the cells, therefore located everywhere in the body. Where there is too much residue, circulation is sluggish, nutritional uptake is poor, and dangerous microbes can release into the bloodstream. The herbs killing off pathogens (a process called die off), can pose a hazard if the connective tissue is overwhelmed with toxins. The Luvos clay absorbs most of the die off and toxins in the intestines and safely eliminates it. Both the *Body High Powder* and the *Major Mineral Mix* are excellent nutritional supplements. Patients who are unable to take various supplements for medical reasons do well on these products because of the pure, non-synthetic, food-based vitamins in flax seed powder that is ground while cold, so it doesn't heat during the process, contributing to spoilage. The *Major Mineral Mix* is a pure liquid mineral supplement that the company refers to as angstrom sized, meaning the mineral is small enough to penetrate the cell wall! Unlike colloidal minerals, they do not require digestion to be broken down into small particles for utilization. The angstrom sized minerals are absorbed into the blood stream within forty-five seconds. A good green food supplement containing spirulina and/or chlorella is highly recommended because of its nutritional content as well as its ability to escort toxins from the body.

As you can see in the protocol, you take the herbal remedy after awakening and getting a start on consuming water for the day. Water is especially important during a cleanse and when taking fiber or clay supplements, because they use more liquid to do their job. Remember not to supplement with fiber or take any form of clay if not having regular bowel movements (at least once a day). If you are not having regular bowel movements, you need to take an herbal laxative. The remedy gets to work, killing parasites, and then comes the Luvos clay to be taken 15-30 minutes later. You do not take fiber supplements or any form of clay with or around the time of taking nutritional supplements because fiber and clay absorb the nutrients and excrete them from the body thereby wasting them. Your nutritional supplements are consumed mid-morning and throughout the day as well as digestive enzymes to assimilate it all! The herbal remedy is taken again 15 minutes before lunch and/or before dinner. Probiotics are taken on an empty stomach before bed; away from herbs that deactivate them. Within the protocol, water is not mentioned but needs to be drunk in between meals and sipped rather slowly. See *Digestion Promoting Rules* and follow the *Vital Food Plan* .

Digestive Health

As a Digestive Health Specialist, I have created a screening you can gauge your digestive health upon and a Symptoms Chart to reference as a guide of digestive complaints. Please call us with any questions or concerns.

Digestive Screening Checklist

NOTE HOW MANY APPLY TO YOU

- ❑ Lack of appetite
- ❑ Excessive appetite
- ❑ Feel hungry shortly after eating a good-sized meal
- ❑ Nausea after meals
- ❑ Sense of fullness with very little food, or delayed 2-4 hrs. after meal (please underline which one)
- ❑ Specific foods upset
- ❑ Swallowing difficulty or frequent choking
- ❑ Burning sensation in the lower portion of chest, especially when lying or bending down
- ❑ Burning or aching relieved by eating
- ❑ Stomach pains or burning 1-4 hrs. after meals
- ❑ Three or more bowel movements in a day
- ❑ Less than one bowel movement (constipation)
- ❑ Difficulty passing stools
- ❑ Small, hard, or dry stools
- ❑ Undigested food in stools
- ❑ Pass mucus in stools
- ❑ Bowel movement shortly after eating (within I hr.)
- ❑ Burping, bloating or gas after eating
- ❑ Lightly colored stools
- ❑ Unexplained itchy skin, especially at night
- ❑ Cracking of heels, or dry flaky skin on feet
- ❑ Easily chill, especially after eating, dizzy when rising, and/or darkness under eyes
- ❑ Loose stools

❑ Consistency or form of stools (e.g., from narrow to lose) changes within the course of the day

If you noted more than three of the above, contact us and let us know. We will target your need for an effective enzyme formula specifically for you.

Add up the following points at the end of the following questions:

Have you had your zinc levels checked in the last 6 months?	
Have taken antibiotics in the last 6 months or for an extended period of time during the last 10 years?	10
Traveled out of the country in the last 10 years?	5
Ever had any type of food allergy / sensitivity testing performed?	10
Have you been diagnosed with any of the following:	
Ulcers – gastric duodenal	10
GERD / Reflux	5
Pancreatitis	10
Celiac Disease	10
IBS / IBD / Colitis	10
Do you take:	
OTC antacids	5
OTC Laxatives / Fiber	5
Prescription medicines for digestion	10

Depending on your total calculated points, you may want to consider our gut restoration program. Contact us to find out more.

Symptoms Chart

Abdominal Complaints:

Symptoms	Possible Cause	Action to Take
Intense pain in the lower right side of the abdomen, possibly starting as a vague pain initially occurring in the epigastric or umbilical region. You may also have nausea, vomiting, or a slight fever.	Appendicitis	Go to an emergency room immediately. Take oregano oil only if not in need of surgery (it thins the blood), or just take one dose. If blood tests show elevated white blood count and surgery is in order, do not allow surgery until appendicitis is confirmed by a CT scan. See Inflammatory Issues below for more... Acupuncture points S25 and S37. Formula Sml containing both Probiotics and enzymes twice daily and enzyme formula TRMA 3x/day for infection.
Severe pain that starts in the upper abdomen and often spreads to the sides and the back. The pain may flare up soon after a large meal, or six to 12 hours after an episode of heavy drinking. You may also have nausea, vomiting, fever, yellowish skin, and a racing heartbeat.	Pancreatitis- see Inflammatory Issues below	Call 911 or go to an emergency room right away. Acute pancreatitis can cause shock, which may result in death if not treated quickly, homeopathic arnica can prevent this. Natural practitioners will check for enzyme deficiencies.
Extremely sharp abdominal pain, perhaps with other acute symptoms. Right side under ribs- spleen (infection) spleen damage or rupture	*Pelvic inflammatory disease *Heart attack *Perforated stomach ulcer *Shock, from allergy *Diabetic emergency *Poisoning	Call 911 or go to an emergency room right away CT scans are helpful in this case.
Pain in upper right side of abdomen; may spread to right upper back, chest, or right shoulder; nausea, vomiting, or gas. Also see below for risks of surgery and alternatives. I have had much success with this and saved many gallbladders!	Gallstones- can be easily removed by the gallbladder protocol or "gallbladder flush" (see below) Ginger tablets help with pain as well as cleanse the blood. Acupuncture or frequency therapy is also effective for the pain during the alternative to surgery!	If this is your first attack, call a doctor for emergency advice. If you can't reach one, go to an emergency room but remember they like to remove organs! Never agree to removal unless a scan/x-ray is done to verify gall stones blocking the duct and elevated white blood counts indicating an emergency due to infection.

In a woman who might be pregnant: severe pain that arises suddenly in the lower right or lower left abdomen, usually without vomiting or fever.	Ectopic pregnancy	Call the doctor for a prompt appointment. If you experience severe abdominal pain or bleeding, call 911 or go to the emergency room right away.
Moderate to severe cramps or occasional cramps that flare up after meals, and vomiting, especially if the vomit smells like stool. Other possible signs include watery or ribbon-like stools, or no stools at all.	Intestinal obstruction	You may want to visit the ER or seek advice from a holistic practitioner. Always treat with herbs for infection. Do bowel cleanse with Luvos clay specifically.
Pain or tenderness in the lower left side of the abdomen, along with fever. You may also have nausea, vomiting, chills, stomach cramps, and either diarrhea or constipation.	Diverticulitis- small pockets or pouches that form in the intestines. It is known that 30% of Americans have it that are over age 60.	See a professional immediately. If you have sharp abdominal pain along with fever, chills, swelling, or nausea and vomiting, call 911 or go to an emergency room right away. You may have peritonitis, a life-threatening infection of the abdominal cavity.
Chronic abdominal pain along with dark urine and yellowish skin and eyes.	Viral hepatitis	See a professional promptly. Take Amino Acid Lysine and herbs for the liver, as well as a homeopathic for immediate results.
Pain in the back that usually spreads under the rib cage, around the front, and into the groin.	Kidney stones	See a professional promptly. Always treat infection with silver and/or herbs. Stop taking calcium until you find out what kind they are.
Searing, stabbing pain in the upper abdomen; pain in the back between the shoulder blades; pain under the right shoulder, and behind the chest bone. Also, may be nausea, vomiting, and indigestion. Gas passing does not relieve pain.	Gall stones or an infection of the gallbladder. They only take 8 hrs. to develop; 90% do not have symptoms! *prevention- do not overeat! Take bile salts under the supervision of a professional trained in such. Lose weight if needed. Drink plenty of water, exercise and consume adequate fiber. Avoid trans fats, chocolate, and carbonated drinks!	If you experience sweating, chills, and fever, see a professional right away. The combination of oregano oil, liquid silver, and performing a LV/GB flush right away is necessary.
Chronic abdominal pain in the upper right quadrant, along with a fever, sore throat, and extreme fatigue.	Mononucleosis or other viral infection	Seek testing. Be sure to get plenty of rest.

Bloody stools or bleeding from the rectum. In some cases, abdominal pain.	Bleeding hemorrhoids, colon polyps, or (rarely) colorectal cancer. (Hemorrhoids and polyps rarely cause abdominal pain.)	Seek medical attention promptly.
In a woman: dull, constant pain in the lower abdomen along with vaginal discharge and fever.	Pelvic inflammatory disease.	Consult your physician for a pelvic exam. Deal with parasites to be assured you do not have a chronic infection. Utilize enzyme therapy.
Dull, gnawing stomach pain that comes and goes. The pain is often worse when the stomach is empty and goes away after eating. You may also have indigestion, nausea, vomiting, heartburn, gas, and dark stools. Dull, gnawing stomach pains that go away when no beverages or food have been consumed for a while = Evaluate dishwashing & dish washer detergent as a cause; remember, nothing rinses off completely! Never use anything on dishes, skin, etc. that you wouldn't eat!	*Stomach ulcer (peptic ulcer) *Gastritis (inflammation of the stomach lining)	Take a ginger glycerite remedy and do our Gut Restoration program. Avoid aspirin, ibuprofen, and other nonsteroidal anti-inflammatory drugs. Do not drink alcohol or smoke. If pain persists or quickly comes back, see your doctor. Call 911 or go an emergency room right away if you throw up blood or anything that looks like coffee grounds; if you feel faint, chilly, or sweaty; if you have black or bloody stools, or if you feel lightheadedness, as if you would faint. If you have sharp back pain with ulcer symptoms; explore other causes as well such as kidney infection.
Frequent burning pain in the upper abdomen or chest, possibly accompanied by a sour taste in the mouth, a lump in the throat, or trouble swallowing.	Gastroesophageal reflux disease (GERD)	Take ginger the first sign of pain. If pain persists or quickly comes back, seek a professional. See your doctor promptly if you have trouble swallowing, especially if solid food gets stuck.
Vague, widespread, cramp-like pain, accompanied by bloating, tiredness, gas, and occasional nausea. You may also have diarrhea, constipation, or bouts of both.	Irritable bowel syndrome	Find ways to reduce stress. Digestive enzymes— under supervision of a trained professional, preferably as directed by a digestive health specialist Heather Holistics). If you have constipation; take aloe and other herbs as well as drink more water. Balance nervous system with essential oil therapy.
Pain in the lower abdomen. You may also have blood or mucus in your stools, fever, unexplained weight loss, skin rashes, tiredness, or joint pain.	Chron's disease (pain in the right side) or ulcerative colitis (with pain in the left side). Dysentery is also a possibility	Consult with a professional promptly. Be sure to tell them if you may be at risk for dysentery, or diarrhea containing blood, which is often caused by exposure to water contaminated by bacteria or protozoa. If diagnosed with ulcerative colitis or Crohn's disease, you should eat nutritious meals, get plenty of rest, and cut back on stress. Avoid alcohol and aspirin.

Pressure in your upper abdomen, especially associated with heartburn.	Hiatal hernia,	Make an appointment with your health care provider. You can also help yourself by avoiding large meals, taking (especially within three hours of bedtime), raising the head of your bed by 4 to 6 inches, and not lying down for three hours after eating.
Pain in the lower abdomen, often combined with burning or stinging when urinating, yellow discharge, difficulty urinating, strong-smelling, murky, or bloody urine; and in women, pain during intercourse	Urinary tract infection	See your doctor promptly. You can help yourself by drinking at least 8 to 10 glasses of water or clear liquids a day. Some physicians advise avoiding alcohol, caffeine, and spicy foods. Don't have intercourse until recovered.
Stomach discomfort or bloating after drinking or eating dairy products, such as cow's milk and ice cream.	Lactose intolerance	Avoid dairy products or take enzymes to help you digest lactose.
Bloating along with fewer than four bowel movements a week, abdominal pain, or hard, dry stools that are difficult to pass.	Constipation	Drink plenty of liquids, take extra magnesium, and walk or exercise each day if possible. If problems persist, call your health care provider for an evaluation. Low thyroid may be a cause.
Sulfur or "rotten egg" smelling burps	H. Pylori or other infection. Celiac Disease (gluten intolerance), too much meat in diet and/ or Lactose intolerance	Eliminate gluten containing grains, avoid dairy products, reduce meat consumption and take enzymes. Treat infection with Olive leaf capsules 3x/day and a tincture of Black walnut, Echinacea, and goldenseal at least 4x/day ideally 15 min. before meals. Do this for the 1st 2 weeks then take tincture 3x/day. Olive leaf can be taken long term and does not counter the friendly flora in gut.
Vomiting	Mostly viral causes although can range from H. Pylori bacterium, to gastritis, poisoning, or brain tumor. Look at food allergies	Evaluate if cause could be viral (is there other flu like symptoms?). Treat as if H. Pylori infection. If vomiting returns periodically, seek a professional.
Abdominal bloating	Stress, poor digestion, infection, disorders such as IBS, Celiac, or lactose intolerance, fatty foods or other enzyme deficiency related disorder. Smoking can also be a cause. Assess for enzyme therapy	Treat as if H. Pylori infection. Consume only homemade soups with limited broth, and veggies. No legumes, dairy, or gluten for at least one week. If symptoms improve, add meat in small amounts. Back into diet. Take food enzymes at every meal and Probiotics first thing in the morning on empty stomach and before going to bed.

Constipation		Dysbosis (imbalance of friendly bacteria in gut), dehydration, infection, or other digestive disorders. Improper diet and deficiencies can be part of the cause.	Sena tea, licorice, Aloe Vera (make smoothies with the whole plant), re-hydrate. See a professional to be evaluated, for further advice, and to direct you on how to use Standard Process products.
Diarrhea	Take clays (Lovos, Bentonite, or activated charcoal). Use a flu homeopathic remedy consisting of Arsenicum alb, Byronia, Eupatorium perf, and Eupatorium up to every 15 min. until symptoms are under control. Then use every 2 hrs. Then 3 times/day until all symptoms are gone. Homeopathic Oscillococcinum is a popular remedy for decreasing duration and intensity of flu symptoms as well (use the same way).		
Food poisoning	Cilantro, Clays to absorb toxins, silver, herbs such as Echinacea, Yarrow, and Elderberry, homeopathic remedies, protoletic enzymes, probiotics every hour on empty stomach for the 1st 4 hrs.		

*More details, patient specific care, professional grade products, and literature may be provided by contacting us.

Homeopathy Tipsheet

I'll provide examples of some homeopathics below to gain a familiarity with how the medicine of homeopathy differs from herbology and other forms of medicine. It is a brilliant and safe system I advise do-it-yourself types to explore.

Homeopathic instructions:

As a general rule of thumb, virtually instant results are obtained if you follow this one simple rule:

~Take remedy 20 minutes away from anything in the mouth.

If you do not receive the expected benefits, take additional action to increase effectiveness:

- Take at least 15-20 minutes prior to any food, drink, cigarettes, gum, etc. (including water), unless otherwise recommended by your health practitioner.
- Take 1 hr. after food.
- Limit raw garlic, onions and other strong spices to one hour after taking homeopathics.
- Limit caffeine and nicotine during homeopathic use
- Mint in any form such as candy, toothpaste, mouthwash, camphor or menthol (as in muscle and joint rubs) and moth balls fumes need to be avoided. They can adversely affect the healing mechanisms of the homeopathic remedy for days.
- Limit exposure to toxins such as paint thinner, cigarette smoke etc. As well as strong orders such as essential oils.
- Place drops under the tongue and hold for 10 seconds to allow for absorption
- Keep homeopathic remedies out of direct sunlight and radiation.

*If you are sensitive to alcohol; dilute dosage in a glass of warm water (3 oz.). Allow one minute from alcohol to evaporate. Or use the pellets or tablets available.

Belladonna: Use when there is a lot of heat with flu symptoms. Sudden fevers, colds, flu, heat conditions, redness, inflammation, throbbing headaches.

Aconitum nap: Frightfulness, shock or anger. It can stop a cold at a sniffle, minimize fever, inflammation.

Bryonia alba: Moody when sick, worse with motion-colds, flu with dry cough; frontal headaches, constipation/nausea.

Cinchona: Recovery and fatigue especially w/ dehydration from flu, diarrhea, vomiting, breast feeding, blood loss.

Nux vom: Chest discomfort with restlessness or chilliness, suffocating cough, fatigue and irritability, especially if stress increased susceptibility.

Whether we call it a cold, flu, hay fever or sinusitis is not important in homeopathy. A combination sinus remedy may suit your cold symptoms better than a remedy called Colds. The key is to find a good fit between the remedy's indications and your symptoms. For example, "Sneezing with a dry burning sensation" is much more telling than "I have a cold." Knowing how to recognize and treat flu symptoms with a homeopathic natural flu remedy will increase the treatment options available to you, and may help you feel better, faster.

Leading a Healing Lifestyle

Heather Holistics helps to facilitate a *healing lifestyle*, and because not everything can be addressed within a single consultation, I find it most effective and convenient to provide handouts of information to cover all the bases.

Considering all aspects of your health includes the substances to which you are exposed. These include household cleaners, your work and living environment such as air and water quality, along with everyday items you may not think about as being harmful.

Preventative medicine is obviously wise and ideal. Visiting a practitioner of natural medicine for advice and check-ups is certainly beneficial. I also believe there are many areas to take control over yourself. With simple changes in the home such as outlined in the *Your Essential Guide for Diet and Nutrition*, you will be gifting yourself a great deal. You set a model of responsibility for your family and others around you.

Keep up the good work!

Always choose all natural cleaning products. Industrial chemicals are unnecessary sources of toxins. Natural products are effective for the intended purposes and health-promoting rather than demoting!

Speaking of clean; hand sanitizers contain dangerous levels of concentrated alcohol (propanol, propyl, or rubbing alcohol), is so dangerous in fact that babies can die within minutes of application! It is easy to make own sanitizer. I would be happy to share the options with you. The form of alcohol used in store bought products causes cancer and is found in many common products you likely use daily, even in food products! Shampoo and body wash, hair styling products, shaving cream, cosmetics, mouthwash, decaffeinated coffee, supplements, carbonated beverages, store-bought fruit juices, cold cereals, and bottled water!

As you are aware, water is a vital piece of the puzzle. Good filtration, even on a decent source of water, can be very helpful in cleaning up avoidable health-hazards. It may not occur to some people that city water is less than ideal. Chlorine and fluoride, both commonly added to water are halogens (a class of highly reactive chemicals). Western Europe and the Netherlands outlawed Floridization after twenty three years of testing. Germany likewise found that the one part-per-million dose recommended is close to that of which long-term use causes damage to humans. Chorine has similar toxic effects as fluoride and again, the U.S. is one of the few countries that persists in dosing public water supplies with both these chemicals.

These highly toxic halogens combine with hydrocarbons to create a carcinogenic effect, are best avoided in your drinking, cooking and bathing water!

For more information see the resources page of my website. Under the *Immune* category you will find *Environmental Factors in Illness*.

Go to VirtualHealthCarePortal.com/store for the above resources

Wellness is more than what you eat! Think about your environment too! What do you clean your home with? How about your daily moisturizer?

1. Air and water quality are very important for the maintenance of a healthy body. HEPA filters are a must for your vacuum and air filter.

2. Lotions, soaps, and other body care products are all loaded with fragrance, preservatives, and other carcinogenic chemicals; even the so-called "All Natural" products. I use pure Aloe Vera toner and facial oil in lieu of lotion. Essential oils added to my facial oil provide a nice addition. Ask for more details and options.

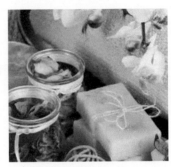

3. Think holistic when it comes to 1st aid needs! Salves and remedies

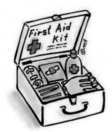

(homeopathic and herbal) are just a phone call away. Heal faster with nature's ingredients.

4. Clean with natural sanitizing and cost effective agents such as vinegar, castile soap and essential oils! Learn more via our workshops and classes!

I'M HAPPY TO ANSWER ANY QUESTIONS YOUH AVE ALONG THEW AY. FEEL FREE TO CALL OR E-MAIL.

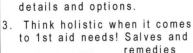

OUR SIGNATURE HOUSEHOLD CLEANER!

HEATHER HOLISTICS NATUROPTHAIC CLINIC

DR. BROOKE HEATHER

CTN HHP, QNT, CBS

(208)231-7149

NATUROPATHICCLINIC.INFO

FIND STORE, BLOG AND RESOURCES ON

VERTRUALHEALTHCAREPORTAL.COM

Nail Indicators of Nutritional Deficiency

Using fingernails (and hands) for diagnosis has been a key part of Oriental medicine. This next section is extremely helpful for any practitioner using nutrition in their practice for it also gives you the signs and symptoms of each deficiency.

Affliction	Related Nutrition and Traditional Chinese Medicine (TMC) Findings
Soft, tear or peel easily, opaque white lines	**PROTEIN**
Dry, brittle, break easily, horizontal or vertical ridges (hypothyroidism may be a contributing factor)	**CALCIUM** TCM medicine asserts that if seen on only the thumbs, investigate excretory system problems. Ridges on all four fingers indicate respiratory weakness or inflammation. Other conditions such as yeast or other infections.
Thin, flat, spoon-shaped, white or yellow nail beds and/or brittle (white nail beds or white coloration near the cuticle with dark coloration near the tip can also indicate chronic liver/kidney disease)	**IRON** TCM medicine says pitting of areas in the nail can mean autoimmune disorders
White spots or bands on nails or nail bed (can also indicate liver/kidney disease or appear consequent of fasting or menstruation)	**ZINC** TCM medicine suggests kidney dysfunction with stripes of white lines presenting horizontally across the nail.
Yellow nail bed, poor or no growth (also indicates possible lymphatic or respiratory congestion)	**VITAMIN E**
Darkened nail beds	**VITAMIN B 12** In TCM medicine, melanoma can be spotted by the appearance of a dark band or streak. If a red or dark line moves with the growing nail and not caused by a local trauma to the nail, it can signal internal bleeding.

Note: Impaired circulation to the extremities, as in Reynaud's phenomenon, phlebitis, etc., can cause any of the above symptoms. Dry, brittle nails can also be caused by excessive exposure to solvents, detergents, nail polish and nail polish remover. Always rule out digestive insufficiency first. See below. The shape of the nails as well as the half-moons indicates additional meanings.

Please allow us in directing you in case-specific care in choosing supplements for best results. The nutrients for which we evaluate your need are food concentrates provided in addition to your diet. Inquire about our Symptom Survey in order to support normal physiology and biochemistry function through Whole Food Targeted Nutrition.

The PH Factor

The measurement of pH is expressed on a scale of 0 to14 and is logarithmic, which means that each step is ten times the previous. In other words, a pH of 4.5 is 10 times more acid than 5.5, 100 times more acid than 6.5 and 1,000 times more acid than 7.5. Water (H_2O) ionizes into hydrogen (H^+) and hydroxyl (OH^-) ions. When these ions are in equal proportions, the pH is a neutral 7. Minerals with a negative electrical charge are attracted to the H^+ ion. These are called acid minerals. Acid minerals include chlorine (Cl^-), sulfur (S^-), phosphorus (P^-), and they form hydrochloric acid (HCl), sulfuric acid (H_2SO_4), and phosphoric acid (H_3PO_4). Minerals with a positive electrical charge are attracted to the negatively charged OH^- ion. These are called alkaline minerals. Nutritionally important alkaline minerals include calcium (Ca^+), potassium (K^+), magnesium (Mg^+), and sodium (Na^+).

Knowing that a reading of 7 is considered neutral, and a solution is considered Acidic when the hydrogen ions (H^+) exceed the hydroxyl ions (OH^-), and a solution is considered Alkaline (base) when the hydroxyl ions (OH^-) exceed hydrogen ions (H^+); the key is to have good ionic concentration in order to maintain a stable pH that fluctuates accordingly, yet stays within ideal range. By eating fresh raw and carefully cooked whole, un-altered whole foods and professional grade supplements, ideal pH is maintained. Abnormal pH is a result of long-term metabolic upset or imbalance. Below I will demonstrate how you can begin to take charge of your health by recording food consumption and pH levels. You will be able to monitor status and recognize when to seek professional help. If pH levels are out of normal range, I encourage you to contact me for further instruction. PH issues and what you do about them must ALWAYS be evaluated in relation to a person's respiratory rate (RR) and breath hold (BH) time. The lungs are initiated to regulate pH on a moment to moment basis. A normal average respiratory rate is 14-18 breaths per minute. If a person, for instance, has a resting RR of 9 breaths per minute, that individual has a potential alkalosis issue. We breathe to blow off acid (having a high breath rate usually results in the blood leaning towards the acid side of normal). If RR is low, the blood leans towards the alkaline side of normal. You should work with a professional that understands this form of testing the metabolism, or I can guide you through it. The body is a complex mechanism and cannot be simply given "alkaline" foods or minerals if pH is found to be "acidic" without the proper evaluation; this is the takeaway in providing the information about pH in relation to RR and BH. For now, you can gain some knowledge from averaging your saliva pH and urinary pH as a preliminary evaluation if you feel things are off with you before you seek the expense of a professional.

Only testing the urine or only testing the saliva pH is not conclusive. The saliva parallels the extracellular fluid (tissue level), thus represents the mineral level in your blood and tissues, unlike the urine. The pH range of urine varies greatly during the day, or should.

NOTE: it is entirely possible to be too alkaline. Many believe the more alkaline the better, focusing solely on the pH of the urine. There is a flip side to everything. Being too alkaline presents its own set of clinical manifestations and needs to be equally addressed, just as you would if you were too acidic.

Recoding the pH

Time	Consumption	SpH	UpH	Feel
6:30		Ideal is 6.4 It should not be below 6.1 5.5 or lower indicates chronic degenerative disease or the groundwork of it.	Depends on what the last meal was. If it was acid forming foods (grains, beans, nuts, and no veggies); ideal pH should range somewhere between 5.8 down to 4.5. This acidic UpH after an acid forming meal means the body has enough alkaline reserves to buffer the acid and the adrenals and kidneys have enough vitality to excrete the metabolic wastes. After such a meal the UpH is 5.8-6.8; the body is barely compensating. The higher the UpH, the worse the buffering system is. In this case the adrenal exhaustion and impaired digestion is present. If also accompanied by a SpH of 5.8- NOT good; the further the pH's are from each other, the worse off you are, and more alkalizing minerals and water are needed.	

An <u>average</u> of 6.4 between the saliva and urine pH is ideal. It is averaged by using the formula below:

(Urine pH _____ + (Saliva pH X 2_____)) / Divided by 3 = _____. This is a quick way to get your averaged PH to determine your general state of health.

Instructions:

Take both urine and saliva pH 2 hours after the AM meal and again 2 hours after your noon meal. Do this for several consecutive days, recording it for record keeping. A "moving pH" is a good thing; it reflects the body's ability to appropriately respond to metabolic acids and remove them!

In general, urine pH should be below 6.5 and saliva pH should be above 6.5. Being consistently alkaline is NOT good! You want the urine pH to move to be acidic in response to the removal of metabolic acids. You do not want to see urine pH above 6.5! 6.1-6.2 is ideal for urine pH.

This is an on-going analysis over the course of two weeks with the purpose of determining how the pH fluctuates throughout the day under different circumstances and food consumption. Use the form provided below or record the five columns onto a notebook for your record keeping.

Ideal Urinary pH 6.1-6.2 (less than 6.1 is acidic and 6.2 or above is alkalosis)

4----------5----------6----------7----------8----------9----------10

Ideal Saliva pH 6.7 (Lower than 6.6 is acidic and 6.7 or above is alkalosis)

An average of 6.4 is ideal (UpH+(SpHx2)/3)

Time	Consumption	SpH	UpH	Feel

Toxicity Questionnaire

0	Rarely or Never Experience the Symptom
1	Occasionally Experience the Symptom- Effect is NOT Severe
2	Occasionally Experience the symptom- Effect is Severe
3	Frequently Experience Symptom- Effect is NOT Severe
4	Frequently Experience- Effect is Severe

1. Digestion

A.	Nausea &/or Vomiting	0 1 2 3 4
B.	Diarrhea	0 1 2 3 4
C.	Constipation	0 1 2 3 4
D.	Bloated feeling	0 1 2 3 4
E.	Belching/Flatulence	0 1 2 3 4
F.	Heartburn	0 1 2 3 4
G.	Tired after eating	0 1 2 3 4

2. Emotions

A.	Mood swings	0 1 2 3 4
B.	Anxiety/Nervousness	0 1 2 3 4
C.	Fearful	0 1 2 3 4
D.	Anger or irritable	0 1 2 3 4
E.	Depression	0 1 2 3 4
F.	Easily overwhelmed	0 1 2 3 4
G.	Poor concentration	0 1 2 3 4
H.	Disinterest or apathy	0 1 2 3 4

Energy/Activity

A.	Fatigue/Sluggishness	0 1 2 3 4
B.	Restless	0 1 2 3 4
C.	Hyperactive	0 1 2 3 4
D.	Insomnia	0 1 2 3 4
E.	Startled awake @ night	0 1 2 3 4

Mind

A.	Poor Memory	0 1 2 3 4
B.	Confusion	0 1 2 3 4
C.	Poor coordination	0 1 2 3 4
D.	Difficulty making decisions	0 1 2 3 4
E.	Slurred speech	0 1 2 3 4
F.	Learning disabilities	0 1 2 3 4

Weight

A.	Cravings	0 1 2 3 4
B.	Compulsive eating	0 1 2 3 4
C.	Over weight	0 1 2 3 4
D.	Weight loss	0 1 2 3 4
E.	Water retention	0 1 2 3 4

Eyes

A.	Watery or itchy	0 1 2 3 4
B.	Swollen/red or sticky	0 1 2 3 4
C.	Dark circles under	0 1 2 3 4
D.	Puffy under eyes	0 1 2 3 4
E.	Sunken in	0 1 2 3 4
F.	Bulging out	0 1 2 3 4
G.	Blurred or tunnel vision	0 1 2 3 4

Ears

A.	Itchy	0 1 2 3 4
B.	Drainage from ears	0 1 2 3 4
C.	Earaches	0 1 2 3 4
D.	Ear infections	0 1 2 3 4
E.	Ringing in ears	0 1 2 3 4
F.	Hearing loss	0 1 2 3 4

Nose

A.	Excessive mucus	0 1 2 3 4
B.	Stuffy	0 1 2 3 4
C.	Hay fever/allergy	0 1 2 3 4
D.	Sneezing attacks	0 1 2 3 4
E.	Chronic sinus prob.	0 1 2 3 4
Page Total		_____

Head

A.	Headaches	0 1 2 3 4
B.	Dizziness	0 1 2 3 4
C.	Faintness	0 1 2 3 4
D.	Pressure	0 1 2 3 4

Lungs

A. Asthma or bronchitis	0 1 2 3 4
B. Shortness of breath	0 1 2 3 4
C. Difficulty breathing	0 1 2 3 4
D. Chest congestion	0 1 2 3 4
E. Pressure/Tightness	0 1 2 3 4

Heart

A.	Chest Pain	0 1 2 3 4
B.	Skipped heart beat	0 1 2 3 4
C.	Rapid heart beat	0 1 2 3 4
D.	Irregular heart beat	0 1 2 3 4
E.	Cold hands &/or feet	0 1 2 3 4

Mouth/Throat

A.	Chronic coughing	0 1 2 3 4
B.	Gag easily	0 1 2 3 4
C.	Need to clear throat	0 1 2 3 4
D.	Canker sores	0 1 2 3 4
E.	Swollen or discolored tough, lips, gums, etc	0 1 2 3 4

Skin/Hair

A.	Excessive sweating	0 1 2 3 4
B.	Moist hands	0 1 2 3 4
C.	Dry skin/hair	0 1 2 3 4
D.	Hair loss	0 1 2 3 4
E.	Acne	0 1 2 3 4
F.	Rashes	0 1 2 3 4
G.	Flushing of face	0 1 2 3 4

Joints/Muscles

A.	Pain or aches in joints	0 1 2 3 4
B.	Pain or aches in musc.	0 1 2 3 4
C.	Feeling of weakness or tiredness	0 1 2 3 4
A.	Burning pain	0 1 2 3 4
B.	Recurrent back aches	0 1 2 3 4
C.	Stiffness or limited movement	0 1 2 3 4
A.	Rheumatoid arthritis	0 1 2 3 4
B.	Osteoporosis	0 1 2 3 4

Other

A.	Frequent infections	0 1 2 3 4
B.	Frequent sickness	0 1 2 3 4
C.	Swollen glands	0 1 2 3 4
D.	Frequent or urgent need to urinate	0 1 2 3 4
E.	Genital itch &/or discharge	0 1 2 3 4

Scoring

* Would benefit from a cleanse

** Definite need to detox

*** Toxic Alert!

Page Total   _____

* Pages 1 & 2 equal 40   *** Pages 1 & 2 over 80

** Pages 1 & 2 equal 60

0	Never	1	Rarely	2	Monthly/Moderately	3	Weekly /Definite Reaction	4	Daily/Sever

Circle the corresponding number based upon your environmental exposure over the last 120 days

Risk or Exposure

A. Frequency of prescription drugs   0 1 2 3 4

    - Side effects are: (Experience side effects but mildly– add 1 point, Side effects are severe–add 3 points)   _____

B. Frequency of over the counter drugs   0 1 2 3 4

C. Do you have adverse reactions to caffeine   0 1 2 3 4

D. Do you develop symptoms upon exposure to fragrance, exhaust, or other chemicals 0 1 2 3 4

E. Do you have a history of significant or frequent exposure to weed spray, insecticides, paint fumes, or any other harsh chemicals?   0 1 2 3 4

Yeast/Candida Evaluation- Short Version

Add the number indicated for each YES answer:

A. Have you taken antibiotics more than once in the past year?....................................35

B. Have you had vaginitis/ prostatitis within the past two years................................20

C. Chronic or persistent urinary tract or vaginal/prostate infections 35

D. Have you taken any form of cortisone type drug for more than two weeks 15

E. Does exposure to new carpet, strong odors, fragrance etc. cause:

    1. Mild reactions 5

    2. moderate to severe symptoms 20

F. Does tobacco smoke really bother you? 10

G. . Have you had athlete's foot, "jock itch", ring worm, or other fungal related infections of the skin or nails?

    1. mild to moderate 10

    2. Persistent or severe 20

H. . Do you crave sugar 10

I. Do you crave breads 10

J. Do you crave alcoholic beverages 10

Enter the rating for each symptom below. **Occasional** or **Mild– 1, Frequent** or **moderately severe– 2, Sever-3**

A. Muscle or joint stiffness, aches, cramps, or soreness for no apparent reason .... _____

B. Feeling "spacey", drained, apathetic, irritable, fidgety, incardinated, moody, etc................ _____

C. Slow to heal, Failing Vision, dizzy .... _____

D. Bad breath, , dry mouth, heart burn, bloating, constipation or diarrhea................ _____

E. Rashes, blisters, bleeding gums, sore or itching throat .... _____

F. Pressure, tightness, or pain in chest, cough, wheezing .... _____

Women Only

A. More than two pregnancies 5

B. Have you taken birth control pills for more than two years 15

Scoring: **40** points– health could **possibly** be effected   **60**– health is **probably** endangered   **90+ – definitely** endangered

Recipes for Resilience

Mineral Milk

Soak raw, unsalted almonds or walnuts overnight in a jar covered with a cloth (1-part almonds to 3 parts purified water). Blend, strain and refrigerate. You can also add some pure vanilla extract to the finished product. Walnuts are superior to other nuts for inflammatory conditions. You can soak organic dried fruit such as raisins with the nuts to add some sweet to your milk, then use the strained material for muffins, pancakes, etc.

Chocolate Mint "Ice-Cream"

Blend a couple ice cubes, a handful of **spinach, a portion of a *banana, a couple drops of peppermint essential oil (Dotera – certified for internal use) and blend. Stir in cacao nibs. **not for Pitta types. * Not for Kapha types.

Sesame Seed Brittle

Melt butter, stir in an equal amount of honey and add *sesame seeds. Spread thin in a glass pan. Let cool before serving. *Not great for Kapha types

Oatdelicious Pancakes

Boil 1 ¼ c. water add 1 ¼ c. Almond Milk (see Mineral Milk)
Soak 1 cup of whole rolled oats in the above with 2 T. honey
After 45 min. of soaking add 2 T. coconut oil and 2 eggs
Combine:

    1 c. spelt, oat or other flour   ½ tsp. sea salt
    2 tsp. Baking Powder

Add to above, stir and cook over oiled griddle and enjoy!

Buckwheat Rye

3 cups buckwheat flour
2 cups whole yogurt

1/2 cup pure water

Mix well and let sit 12-24 hrs.– this allows for the enzymes to be released making it superior to today's bread!

Add:
3 large eggs
2 T. oil
1/3 cup agave/molasses mixture or 1/3 cup maple syrup

1 tsp. sea salt
2 tsp. baking soda
1 tsp. dill
2 tsp. Caraway seeds

Scones

3 c. rice flour
1 c. butter

1 c. plain yogurt

Mix thoroughly in a glass bowl then set covered with a clean towel 6-12 hours at room temperature.

Stir in about ½ tsp. baking powder. Add a couple tablespoons sugar or sweetener of choice, vanilla extract and a dash of salt. *Optional*: Fold in dried fruit.

Make a long roll, flatten to about ½ inch thickness and cut triangles. Bake at 350° till turning golden brown.

These below are called "meal ideas" due to the following not having specific measurements, rather approximations; just as you would making stir-cooked meals – you eyeball it.

Meal Ideas

Medicinal Curry

Make basmati rice

Mix one bunch cilantro with one can coconut milk in a food processor or blender for a raw green sauce to top it all

Sauté mushrooms (maitake, Shitake and/or regular), with fresh garlic, onions and ginger. Sprinkle curry powder on mushrooms but make your own and eliminate peppers (nightshades) if inflammation is an issue!

Curry: Turmeric, Ginger, Cloves,
Cinnamon, Coriander, Allspice, cumin,
fenugreek, mustard, red pepper

Add rice to curry/mushrooms, mix well. Top with green sauce and raw cashews

Cashew Curry Sauce With "Noodles"

1 Bunch Cilantro
½ cup cashew butter
1 T. lemon

1 T. Vinegar
4 garlic cloves

Mix in blender and top "noodles" (zucchini shreds)

Hearty Healthy Tai Soup

1 T. Oil
3 Garlic Cloves, Minced\
2-6 oz. Boneless, Skinless Chicken
Breasts, chopped
1/2 tsp. Turmeric
1/4 tsp. Hot Chili Powder
2 T – ½ c Creamed Coconut
4 cups Broth (Veggie)

2 T. Lemon or Lime Juice
2 T. Crunchy Peanut Butter
12 oz. Thread Egg Noodles, broken
into small pieces
1 T. Finely Chopped Spring Onion
1 T. Chopped Fresh Coriander
Salt and Pepper to taste

1---Heat oil and fry garlic for 1 min. until golden.
Add chicken, Turmeric and Chili powder and stir-fry for 3-4 min.

2---Crumble the creamed coconut into hot broth and stir until dissolved.
Pour onto the chicken and add the lemon or lime juice, Peanut Butter and Egg Noodles.

3---Cover and simmer for about 15 min. Add the spring onion and coriander, then season well and cook another 5 min.

Healing Chicken Ginger Soup

If you would like to use a whole chicken for this soup instead of the two chicken breasts, simply double the ingredients for the broth and the soup and use an 8 or 12-quart pot instead. Be sure to add the rice noodles to each individual bowl if you plan to have leftovers. Adding them to the whole pot and then reheating the soup the next day can cause the noodles to get quite mushy. This soup also freezes very well, just don't add the noodles or the raw toppings to your freezable portions. Fresh Thai chilies and lemongrass can be found at places like Whole Foods or at your local Asian Market.

For the Broth:
2 bone-in organic chicken breasts
(about 2 pounds total)
8 cups water

1 large onion, chopped
3 stalks celery, chopped
1 large carrot, chopped

1 whole head garlic, cut in half crosswise
1/4 to 1/2 cup finely chopped fresh ginger (or more!)
2 to 3 Thai chilies, chopped or 1 teaspoon crushed red chili flakes

2 cups chopped shiitake mushrooms
1 stalk fresh lemongrass, chopped cilantro stems
1 teaspoon whole black peppercorns
3 teaspoons Herbamare or sea salt

For the Soup:
1 medium onion, cut into crescent moons
3 to 4 stalks celery, sliced into diagonals
3 carrots, cut into matchsticks

2 to 3 cups sliced shiitake mushrooms
cooked chicken pulled from the bone and chopped
sea salt and freshly ground black pepper to taste

Optional Additions/Toppings:
rice noodles
chopped fresh basil
chopped fresh Napa cabbage

chopped fresh cilantro
chopped fresh Thai green chilies
lime wedges

To make the broth, place all ingredients for broth into a 6-quart pot. Cover and bring to a boil, reduce heat medium-low and simmer for 1 1/2 to 2 hours. Strain broth into a large bowl or another pot using a colander. Place chicken breasts onto a plate to cool. Pour the broth back into the pot. Once chicken is cooled, remove the skin, pull the meat from the bone and chop the chicken into bite-sized pieces.

Place all the veggies for the soup (onion, carrot, celery, and shiitake mushrooms) into the pot with the broth. Cover and simmer for about 15 to 20 minutes. Add the chicken. Season with salt and pepper to taste. Simmer a minute or two more or until vegetables are cooked to your liking. Ladle soup into bowls and serve with a handful of basil, cilantro, and cabbage on top. Sprinkle with Thai chilies if desired.

Look up Bieler's Broth as a staple to utilize in soups and other dishes as well as the "cold remedy" as traditionally used and now called "chicken broth." Note that tetra pack or canned broth does NOT contain the healing attributes that bone broth does, also referred to as mineral broth. Today's version of "chicken broth" made with bouillon is not a healing food either, in fact it is quite the opposite.

Lacto fermented vegetables

These provide a viable source of probiotics (at a cost well below most supplements) to heal and maintain a healthy gut. These beneficial microorganisms attach to receptors in our guts sending a signal to the immune system that says, "everything is okay, no need to overreact to foods and other things entering the gut, let's keep everything calm." If you are dealing with multiple allergies, chances are your gut is out of balance and needs a daily dose of beneficial microorganisms. These crispy, sour, salty vegetables are highly addicting and an easy, economical way to maintain a healthy gut.

Getting Started
1 glass quart jar with a plastic lid
1 to 1 1/2 tablespoons sea salt

2 cups filtered water

Any Combination of Raw Organic Vegetables:

Cauliflower
Beets
Carrots

Bell Peppers
Green Beans
Cabbage

Make sure contents are covered with water (pound down into jar). You can add juiced celery (high in sodium). You may wish to speed up the process with a starter culture, such as kefir grains, whey, or commercial starter powder. A kraut pounder tool can be helpful to pack the jar and eliminate any air pockets. Seal the jar and store in a warm, slightly moist place for 24 to 96 hours, depending on the food being cultured. Ideal temperature range is 68-75 degrees Fahrenheit. Remember, heat kills the microbes! Refrigerate to slow down the fermentation process.

Topping salads with lacto-fermented foods is a great way to sneak it into your diet or that of your family's!

High Octane Vegetable Dip and Sauce

Combine any proportion of the following in a glass jar to soak in water 8 hours:

Almonds, sunflower and pumpkin seeds. Strain water and place in a high-powered blender, such as a Vitamix, with water, brewer's yeast and Liquid Aminos. This can be made thick for a dip (my favorite vegetable to pair with it is broccoli), or thinner for a salad dressing. You may also wish to spice it up adding curry seasoning or jalapeños and cilantro.

Ranch Dressing

Combine equal amounts of heavy cream with buttermilk, stir with a wooden spoon or silicone spatula, cover with cheese cloth or a clean kitchen towel and let set at room temperature for 6-10 hours (depending on temperature). Add salt, garlic powder, onion flakes and dill to taste. Just a pinch of Xanthan gum thickens the dressing. Simply blend or shake jar to congeal the dressing. Keep refrigerated after seasoned.

Other resources:

- The Weston A. Price Foundation (202)3634394 shoppingguide@westonaprice.org
- Dr.Mercola.com a wealth of information in newsletters. Sign up and be informed!
- *Nourishing Traditions* by Sally Fallon (book with recipes)
- *The New Natural Healing* Cookbook by Bessie Jo Tillman

Products:

https://www.virtualhealthcareportal.com/endorsed-products.html